ATTACHMENTS TO WAR

NEXT WAVE: NEW DIRECTIONS IN WOMEN'S STUDIES

A series edited by Inderpal Grewal, Caren Kaplan, and Robyn Wiegman

ATTACHMENTS TO WAR

BIOMEDICAL LOGICS AND VIOLENCE IN
TWENTY-FIRST-CENTURY AMERICA

JENNIFER TERRY

DUKE UNIVERSITY PRESS / *Durham and London* / 2017

© 2017 Duke University Press
Printed in the United States of America on acid-free
paper ♾
Designed by Matthew Tauch
Typeset in Chaparral Pro and ITC Officina Sans Std
by Graphic Composition, Inc., Bogart, Georgia

Library of Congress Cataloging-in-Publication Data
Names: Terry, Jennifer, [date] author.
Title: Attachments to war : biomedical logics and
violence in twenty-first-century America / Jennifer
Terry.
Other titles: Next wave.
Description: Durham : Duke University Press, 2017. |
Series: Next wave : new directions in women's studies |
Includes bibliographical references and index.
Identifiers: LCCN 2017013529
ISBN 9780822369684 (hardcover : alk. paper)
ISBN 9780822369806 (pbk. : alk. paper)
ISBN 9780822372806 (ebook)
Subjects: LCSH: United States—History, Military—21st
century. | War—Medical aspects—History—21st
century. | Regenerative medicine—United States—
History—21st century. | Prosthesis—United States—
History—21st century. | Medical microbiology—
United States—History—21st century.
Classification: LCC E897.T47 2017 | DDC
355.009730905—dc23
LC record available at https://lccn.loc.gov
/2017013529

Cover art: Daniel Arsham, *White Selenite Eroded
Holding Hands*, 2015. Selenite, hydrostone, 17 × 14 ×
5 in. (43.2 × 35.6 × 12.7 cm). Image courtesy of the
artist and Galerie Perrotin, New York.

Duke University Press gratefully acknowledges
the support of the UCI Humanities Commons at
University of California, Irvine, which provided funds
toward the publication of this book.

FOR SURINA

who has taught me many truths
about living and loving well

CONTENTS

ABBREVIATIONS

ACEP	Army Center for Enhanced Performance
AFIRM	Armed Forces Institute of Regenerative Medicine
AMA	American Medical Association
AVA	Anthrax Vaccine Adsorbed
AVIP	Anthrax Vaccine Immunization Program
BARDA	Biomedical Advanced Research and Development Authority
BMI	brain-machine interface
BPHS	Basic Package of Health Services
BTWC	Biological and Toxin Weapons Convention
CBRN	chemical, biological, radiological, and nuclear weapons
CDC	Centers for Disease Control and Prevention
COIN	counterinsurgency
CPA	Coalition Provisional Authority
CSH	combat support hospital
DARPA	Defense Advanced Research Projects Agency
DCBI	dismounted complex blast injury
DHS	Department of Homeland Security
DoD	Department of Defense
DWB	Doctors without Borders
ECM	extracellular matrix
EPA	Environmental Protection Agency
EPHS	Essential Package of Hospital Services
FDA	Food and Drug Administration
FET	Female Engagement Teams
HHS	Department of Health and Human Services

HMO	health maintenance organization
IED	improvised explosive device
IMF	International Monetary Fund
IVAW	Iraq Veterans Against the War
MBPI	Michigan Biologic Products Institute
MSF	Médecins sans Frontières (Doctors without Borders)
NATO	North Atlantic Treaty Organization
NBACC	National Biodefense Analysis and Countermeasures Center
NGO	nongovernmental organization
NIH	National Institutes of Health
NPR	National Public Radio
NSF	National Science Foundation
OEF	Operation Enduring Freedom (Afghanistan, October 7, 2001–December 28, 2014)
OIF	Operation Iraqi Freedom (Iraq, March 19, 2003–August 31, 2010)
OND	Operation New Dawn (Iraq, September 1, 2010–December 15, 2011)
PTSD	posttraumatic stress disorder
RIC	Rehabilitation Institute of Chicago
RP	Revolutionizing Prosthetics
SCIF	Sensitive Compartmented Information Facility
TATRC	U.S. Army Telemedicine and Advanced Technology Research Center
TBI	traumatic brain injury
TMT	Transformational Medical Technologies Initiative
USAID	U.S. Agency for International Development
USAMRMC	U.S. Army Medical Research and Materiel Command
VA	Veterans Administration
WHO	World Health Organization
WILPF	Women's International League for Peace and Freedom
WMD	weapons of mass destruction
WSP	Women Strike for Peace

ACKNOWLEDGMENTS

The most satisfying part of writing a book is thanking the many people who enabled me to write it.

Thanks to Courtney Berger at Duke University Press for her intelligence and care in guiding this project toward its completion and to Sandra Korn, Liz Smith, and Christine Riggio for their editorial and artistic assistance. I owe a debt of gratitude to the two anonymous reviewers of the manuscript, whose comments and suggestions vastly improved the book. Thanks also to I-Lien Tsay and Heather Murray for their research assistance in the early stages of this project.

For taking the time to read or listen to parts of the manuscript and then providing valuable comments, I am grateful to Caren Kaplan, Inderpal Grewal, Laura Hyun-Yi Kang, Michelle Murphy, Lisa Cartwright, Emma Heaney, Laleh Khalili, Deborah Cowen, Elizabeth F. S. Roberts, Minoo Moallem, Kristen Peterson, Mara Mills, A. B. Huber, José Esteban Muñoz, Tavia Nyong'o, Rayna Rapp, Ann Pelligrini, Deborah Cohler, Raegan Kelly, Karen Tongson, Ken Wissoker, Tara McPherson, Steve Anderson, Kathryn Lofton, H. M. Lukes, Jake Kosek, Sima Shakhsari, Elora Shehabuddin, Jennifer Hamilton, Banu Subramaniam, Angela Willey, Khary Polk, Lynn Morgan, Laura Briggs, Gary Wilder, Nadia Abu El-Haj, Alondra Nelson, Rebecca Jordan-Young, Christine Ehrick, Zöe Wool, Sasha Sabherwal, Thyrza Goodeve, Anitra Grisales, J. V. Fuqua, Lucy Suchman, Toby Beauchamp, Liz Montegary, Aaron Belkin, Abigail Boggs, Laura Wexler, Amy Kaplan, Jeanne Scheper, Lilith Mahmud, Catherine Sameh, Emily Thuma, Kimberly Icreverzi, Kimberly Feig, Ari Laskin, Robyn Wiegman, Rebecca L. Stein, Thea Cacchioni, Candace Moore, Elizabeth Reis, and Tim Seiber.

The project was cultivated in the context of various working groups, seminars, and intellectual communities, including the University of California Working Group on Militarism in Everyday Life (organized by Caren

Kaplan and Minoo Moallem) and the UC Working Group on Cultures of Militarization (organized by Caren Kaplan). I am grateful to fellow members of the Working Collective on Geographies of Conflict and Intervention at UC Irvine, Anna Zagos, Leah Zani, and Padma Govindan, for our many discussions about this and related projects. From my seminar on Feminism, Conflict, and Humanitarianism at UC Irvine I especially thank Stefanie Lira, Jessica Pruett, Valentina Ricci, Benjamin Kruger-Robbins, and Megan Zane for helping me think through important issues. And from the seminar on Gender and Militarization at Columbia University, I thank Feride Eralp and Isabel Peñaranda for our conversations. I also thank the many generations of former students at Berkeley, Columbia, Ohio State, and UC Irvine who have inspired me along the way to complete this book.

A vast network of caring friends and kin helped sustain me through the process of research and writing. Thanks especially to Laura Hyun-Yi Kang, Caren Kaplan and Eric Smoodin, Inderpal Grewal and Alfred Jessel, Jo-Ann and Katherine Acey, James Gallagher and Matthew Pealer, Lisa Cartwright, L. B. Johnson, Marcia M. Gallo and Ann Cammett, Arnel Laxamana, Rey Pascual, Evan Wilder, Sharon Ullman, B. Ruby Rich, Patricia White and Cynthia Schneider, Polly Thistlethwaite and Liz Snyder, Joy Fuqua, Christina Crosby and Janet Jakobsen, Emma Heaney, Damon Northrup and Jessica Davies, Christine Balance, Alexandra Vazquez, Kim Gerrard, Heather Lukes and Molly McGarry, Evelyn Dulce-del Villar, Javid Syed and Michael Simonson, Daniel Lee, Huy Le, Stephen Marley, David J. Thomas, Will Guerra and Andrew Parsons, Brian Freeman and Peter Stein, Julie Nice, Kris Peterson, James Renteria, Kathleen Irvine and Jim Danno, Deborah Cowen, Laleh Khalili, Elizabeth Reis, Catherine Sameh, Arlene Keizer, Thyrza Goodeve, Karen Bermann, and the Sanchez family, especially Diane. I also want to acknowledge members of my extended family, who have been with me through the writing. Thanks to Dane Terry and Merisa Bissinger, Neal Terry and Henry Rasu, Fazilet Khan-O'Flynn and Seamus O'Flynn, Akbar and Abbas Khan, Naveed Irfani, Muneeza Ayaz Irfani and Mehrunisa Ayaz, Ayaz Ahmed Khan and Zarina Ayaz Khan, Asad Khan and Harma Hartouni and their wonderful children, Zeus, Xena, and Petra.

I want to acknowledge and remember my father, Richard Terry, who left this planet many years ago, and my mother, Patricia Herr Terry, who passed away during the time I was working on this book. Both devoted their lives to public service, both had a deep love of learning, and both were committed to making the world a place of justice and peace. I thank them for the moral guidance and opportunities they gave me.

My deepest gratitude goes to Surina Khan for all the love, affection, and life adventures we have shared. And here is a final shout-out to Rosie, our dog, for coming along for the ride.

Introduction

BEING ATTACHED

My father was a soldier in the U.S. Army. He died of brain cancer in a VA hospital on Memorial Day in 1977 at the age of forty-nine. In 1944, in order to enlist at seventeen, he told a recruiter he was eighteen. It was a way out of a rough childhood of poverty and neglect. He was trained in the Signal Corps and served in World War II and the Korean War. After he and my mother married and had my two older brothers and me, he was deployed to Vietnam for two tours of duty, one in 1964–65 and the other in 1970–71. He assumed the duties of supply sergeant and helicopter gunner. He sustained serious head injuries during each tour, first by grenade shrapnel in a nighttime attack that killed eight American soldiers and wounded over a hundred more, and the second by a group of GIs who attacked him on his way back to his barracks after cashing his monthly paycheck, "leaving him for dead," as my mother put it. There might have been drugs involved in this second incident. The story was told to us in a cryptic fashion.

  When my father was away, I prayed each night at bedtime to someone called "God" for two things: that my father would not be killed so that he could return home to us and that, when he returned, he would stop drinking so that the fits of rage would end. By twelve I had learned from witnessing the terrible toll war took on my father that among those Americans who most abhor war are the ones who return home from fighting them. Next in line are their loved ones. I also learned that many of the leaders who declare war avoid actually putting their own bodies on the line. In time I came to see my childlike and provincial realizations as woefully myopic. Learning the history of U.S. imperialism, I recognized that I was implicated in war as a citizen of a superpower responsible for using armed conflict to seize control of resources and exert its influence all over the world.

For many years I considered the question of whether it is possible for Americans to meaningfully and materially oppose war when its entanglements are so diffuse and deeply rooted in the very fabric of life in this country. My personal history as it relates to this central question motivated me to write this book. I started the research for it in the first decade of the twenty-first century, spurred by the two massive war mobilizations undertaken, first in 2002 in Afghanistan and then in 2003 in Iraq, by the administration of President George W. Bush with the support of a majority of members of the U.S. Congress and in coalition with our NATO allies. In the book I focus on the period bracketed by these officially declared wars but also note that the tactics, logics, and tools of domestic policing are increasingly appropriated from military operations and that war, in this sense, is now never-ending and pervasive. An additional twist is that the wars waged in Afghanistan and Iraq were rationalized by our government as necessary and beneficial to the inhabitants of those regions. They would "liberate" ordinary people from tyranny and help "cultivate" free-market capitalism (often used interchangeably with *democracy*) in those places. Though also staged as urgent operations for securing America from "terrorism," a cloying rhetoric of beneficence saturated much of the U.S. pro-war discourse in these early decades of the century. We were promised that the wars would be efficient and rapidly resolved, surgical in their precision. In the words of Bush's vice president, "We will, in fact, be greeted as liberators."[1] Regime change would swiftly be followed by "nation-building." The invasions were fueled by fantasies of technoscientific precision symbolized by a massive arsenal of sophisticated weapons systems and elaborate logistical protocols according to which only the blameful "terrorists" would be killed. Alongside nationalist rhetoric of protecting the United States, perverse claims about care and compassion were part of the ideological mystification aimed at acquiring the support of the American public for these large-scale offensives. It was not always an easy sell, especially after the wars dragged on and the nation-building plans were exposed as corrupt, rife with sectarian antagonisms, and jackpots for war profiteers overcharging taxpayers through their private contracting firms. A central concern of mine in this book is to track how "care" operated in the rhetoric of pro-war officials and, more specifically, to analyze how it tied wars of this sort to biomedical logics in the actual treatment of (some and not other) wounded bodies as well as in the execution of war itself.

Without a doubt there are organizations and people in the United States who are opposed to war and who question the massive amount of resources that are dedicated to weapons development, policing operations, and overseas military deployments. Others are hawkish proponents of war, seeing in it many opportunities for demonstrating hypermasculine force, acquiring resources, controlling territory, making profits, and exerting political power at home and abroad. Many others remain conveniently unaware of the depth and reach of the nation's commitment to war and militarization, comfortably protected from war's more obvious realities because they are not required to fight, even as they may materially benefit from it. Complex entanglements whose origins can be traced back to the European conquest of the Americas attach us to war not only in visibly apparent ways but in subtle and insidious ways as well. In this book I examine the realm of biomedicine and of biomedical logics as these entangle Americans in war. I have chosen this focus because biomedicine participates in rationalizing our recent wars that are fought not only in the name of national defense but also in the name of an abstraction called "humanity." Technoscientific fantasies of miraculous healing and of "humane" war-fighting entangle violence with dreams of surpassing bodily limitations and of performing antiseptic death. Biopolitics meets necropolitics: laws and policies aimed at maximizing the bodily potential of the population while managing risks are intertwined with laws and policies in which killing or neglecting unto death together make up how "society must be defended."[2]

I use the neologism *biomedicine* to encompass the multiplying branches of modern biological sciences in their convergence with medical research, treatment, and profiteering. *Biomedical logics* are ways of reasoning that manifest in discourses, representations, narratives, and practices animated by the idea of *care*. Biomedical logics, I argue, interweave with neoliberal ideals that promise freedom, democracy, prosperity, and self-improvement while also lending a strange valence to war, one that sees in highly technical violence the hope of rehabilitation, regeneration, security, and the development of humane tactics for waging war. Biomedicine can serve to make excuses for violence, whether these excuses come in the form of knowledge that can be acquired through research on wounds and diseases or in the form of claiming that war can be carried out in efficient targeting in which only the blameful will be violated.

I analyze the dynamics and mediations of several key examples of biomedical projects dealing with war in order to take issue with recent state-sponsored violence carried out overseas and sometimes tested on disempowered communities at home. My argument is that for citizens of the United States to meaningfully oppose war requires gaining an understanding of how our attachments to it are embedded in everyday life and institutionalized in and beyond government in the interwoven industries of media, biotechnology, finance, and higher education.[3] *Attachments to War* provides examples of these entanglements by examining the manifest promises about the future that are evident in our enchantment with biomedicine. The intended audience encompasses readers of any political sensibility, but I especially seek to reach those who are critical of U.S. militarized adventures of the twenty-first century—at home and abroad—but who may benefit from further examination and questioning of the great existential effects of our empire's entanglement with languages and practices associated with care and healing, an entanglement that has too frequently made violence a natural (though tragic) process rather than a political project into which a meaningful intervention can be made.

SCOPE OF THE BOOK

Following a contextualizing chapter on the nexus of war and biomedical logics, I focus in depth on three main areas of biomedical research: diagnosis and treatment of war-generated polytrauma, postinjury bionic prosthetics design, and the cultivation of infectious pathogens rationalized as defense projects. I zero in on developments that occurred between 2002 and 2014, when the United States was officially engaged in combat operations in Afghanistan and Iraq. The book took shape as many of the events I describe were unfolding. We know that despite President Barack Obama's formal announcement in October 2011 ending the war in Iraq and another, made in December 2014, ending the combat mission in Afghanistan, conflict continued in the form of U.S.-led special operations raids, drone strikes, and security-detention operations not only in those regions but in many locations around the world. The nation's surveillance activities proliferated at home and abroad as part of an ever-vigilant anticipation of terrorist attacks. War persisted even as it transmogrified and was mystified by new technologies, covert tactics, and ideologies of security. I realize there is an arbitrary quality to any periodization, but delimiting the chronological scope was necessary in order to finish the book. Where relevant, I have incorporated historical material that preceded 2002. I examine a selection of products and therapies to treat war-wounded men and women, chiefly stem cell–derived tissue cultivation for polytrauma patients (chapter 2), bionic limbs programmed with artificial intelligence that are designed for amputees (chapter 3), and antibiotic/antiviral agents aimed at engineering immunities in the context of infectious disease and biowarfare (chapter 4). The book could have been much longer, bringing into its frame other examples of how biomedicine, war making, and financial speculation are entangled—for example, in the production of treatments for war-generated psychological distress, as well as the use and abuse of biopsychological tools for enacting torture in interrogations at secret detention sites. I have opted for a selective focus rather than a comprehensive survey. If it succeeds in its aim, *Attachments to War* will provide ideas to further our understanding of how war and biomedicine are bound together and for loosening these bonds to make way for ethical futures.

The book focuses on developments in the U.S. military and security apparatus, its biomedical industry, its media stories, and its citizens' behavior. Each of these operates in transnational circuits.[4] America is a key formation where the convergence of money, military power, and medical science draws experts and investors to perceived opportunities facilitated by certain transnational networks that are involved in one way or another in the mutual provocation between war making and biomedical knowledge production. *Attachments to War* focuses on the war politics of biomedicine—the power-laden nexus entangling war and biomedicine— in the United States, the country that until 2014 spent more on its military than the next biggest countries of the world combined and has the most expensive health care in the world.[5] America, however, is not a sealed-off location; far from it. Developments here are subject to global and transnational dynamics, including media products that travel across borders as well as fluctuations in currency rates and stock exchanges, conflicts over resource extraction, and massive social dislocations caused by armed conflict, environmental disasters, and capital flight. *Attachments to War* zeroes in on the ideologies and practices that account for America's highly militarized character as it relates to an enchantment with biomedicine.

Whose bodies are recognized for their sacrifice when it comes to the knowledge acquired through treating the wounded? By what means are they recognized? Whose wounds signify the debt a nation owes? And whose do not? In the book's case-study chapters we encounter patients, their families and friends, physicians, therapists, engineers, scientists, military strategists, bureaucrats, lab administrators, motivational speakers, advertisers, and investors who populate the narratives of biomedical promise put forth by major newspapers, business magazines, television news shows, TED Talks, biomedical advertising, and military public relations offices. These persons and bodies interact with the concept of *biomedical salvation* in a variety of different, unequal, and contradictory ways.

No actor in the biomedicine-war nexus is categorically lionized or demonized in this book. Instead I frame the book as an inquiry into the dynamic field of discourses, practices, and institutions that entangle people differently, depending on a variety of factors and their location in relation to the interwoven social technologies of profession, nationality, socioeconomic class, race, and gender. In this dynamic field notions of potency derive from the injuries caused by evolving types of weapons and strategies of force, drawing vitality, morbidity, and mortality into close contact. This is an existential reality, experienced in different ways, and an aporia that I seek to understand.

War and medicine are in a relationship of mutual provocation whereby new forms of wounding and illness generate biomedical knowledge and vice versa. I contend that this relationship of provocation perpetuates and elaborates processes of militarization through which war comes to be tacitly accepted as a necessary condition for human advancement. I engage critically with the work of scholars who have asked how and why modern wars are fought in the name of humanity. I examine the calculated costs and benefits that influence medical decisions about whose bodies should be cared for and whose are considered expendable in recent officially declared wars America launched in coalition with its allies. I draw upon the conceptual work of other scholars and my own close analysis of an array of cultural objects, actors, narratives, institutions, technologies, and processes that make promissory gestures about the future of life. These gestures sell new medical technologies as investment portfolios in various contexts of speculation that are animated by ongoing and anticipated armed conflict.

Acts of wounding provoke the expansion of medical knowledge.[6] Devastating physical trauma caused by improvised explosive devices can be survived now, thanks to advanced blood-clotting products and rapid emergency evacuation procedures. Mangled and destroyed limbs resulting from high-powered detonations offer the occasion for building bionic devices that rely on artificial intelligence to ambulate the survivor. Deadly and rapidly mutating pathogens developed as weapons provide the impetus for massive research funding to develop "medical countermeasures," which are themselves part of a growing and terrifying arsenal, engineered through recombinant genomic science. A *destroy-and-build* logic is evident in new weapons systems that maim bodies, that are then subject to extreme medical interventions, regeneration therapies, and bodily enhancement. I focus on narratives and representations related to research done by physicians and scientists working at the forefront of the medical biotechnology industry rather than on clinical practice. The industry is highly speculative and financially risky because it often takes many years to bring a device or treatment to the market, and many of the treatments fail in clinical trials. Government contracts awarded to biotechnological and pharmaceutical companies helped to infuse this troubled sector of the economy with bountiful funding. This is why *biomedical war profiteering* is a leitmotif that appears throughout the book.

METHODS

The medical industry and the U.S. military have a long and storied relationship. From smallpox blankets to titanium limbs, their connection is enduring. As Michel Foucault noted, the genius of medicine was to make itself look apolitical, which made it all the more political.[7] Biomedical logics are neither politically neutral nor aligned with any particular political perspective. Instead, I argue, they can be enlisted to serve a range of political agendas. *Attachments to War* is an iteration of some of the specific, and sometimes horrible, ways that war-generated medicine continues to naturalize the notion that biomedicine and war are separate spheres, that the former is apolitical, and that care and violence oppose one another. I argue that biomedical logics are constitutive of the culture of the Global War on Terror, but they are seldom recognized as such. Thus a key method of the book involves taking a look at what is hiding in plain sight.

War is a highly mediated process, especially in the twenty-first century. Many of the hundreds of primary sources I analyze in this book are corporate broadcast and print media material or from offices of the U.S. military that are highly attuned to the significance of appealing to the public for support of the nation's imperial goals. In these materials war is presented through particular narrative conventions and visual representations that rehearse an enduring claim of Total War societies like ours: war is hell, we are reminded, but it yields important knowledge for the future.

Throughout the book I rely on conceptual approaches and methods drawn from cultural studies and feminist science studies. Cultural studies maps how power and knowledge come together, or rather how power-knowledge materializes in thoughts, ideas, images, identities, products, and relations. Cultural studies foregrounds critical reflection on the production of meaning, assuming culture to be constituted through dynamics of difference rather than being a homogeneous or static entity. Culture is a contested terrain, to paraphrase the field's founder, Stuart Hall.[8] Conflicts over meaning involve social subjects—individual people and other agents of social relations (such as universities, governments, religious congregations, corporations, militaries, families, etc.)—and changing (sometimes unpredictable) systems of signification. These conflicts may be more visible in the context of crisis. In the case of the mediated sources I analyze, the crisis stemmed, in part, from the increasingly unpopular wars in Iraq and Afghanistan waged on what became generally regarded as either insufficient, discrepant, or downright false pretenses. I seek to show that narrative presentations pertaining to these wars are in the grain of other popular entertainments that indeed serve to make the violence of war something we have already incorporated into daily life and bodily practice, but of whose many effects we remain disturbingly unaware.

I attempt to break through some of the disciplinary boundaries that function to maintain control over who gets to talk about war, foreign policy, and military operations. The disciplines of political science, military history, and international relations have claimed special authority over these matters. Very little of the writing in these fields has paid attention to critical scholarship that has emerged from feminist studies, ethnic studies, and disability studies. Through an eclectic theoretical mapping of the central problem of the book and through deliberately eccentric citational practices, I seek to enact and embed a kind of critical intervention in how war is considered in the hegemonic disciplines that have laid claim to being its primary interpreters. I also seek to break the hold that military historians have had on the place of medicine and medical knowledge in the history of modern warfare. Where relevant, I focus on the identity categories pertaining to the stratified power relations of gender, race, class, and sexuality. But the book is less about identity formation and more about interrogating the conditions under which power is generated by epistemological systems that produce habits of thinking about how war and medicine are generally understood—how these two formations come to be naturalized.

Biomedical science is an object of critical scrutiny in *Attachments to War*. I draw on methods from feminist science studies to look critically at science in context, noting how history, politics, and economics influence scientific practice, from grant writing and laboratory research to the publishing of findings and their application in the world. Ruth Hubbard argues that science is a social enterprise and that for every fact there is a factor—a person or persons responsible for establishing the fact. Scientific laws and the facts of science, she notes, reflect the interests of the university-educated, economically privileged, predominantly white men who have produced them. The ideas, institutional priorities, professional networks, and funding sources that are available to this elite group play central roles in what kind of research is undertaken, who is allowed to undertake it, and what applications it will generate. Feminist science studies further recognizes what Hubbard refers to as "the indispensable unity of subjectivity and objectivity in every act of knowing": that the pretense of pure objectivity serves to disguise ideological presumptions that are embedded in scientific research and allows researchers to remain unaccountable for the partial perspective they inevitably have.[9]

The research and analysis I present aspire to the sort of analytical work that Donna Haraway called for in her critical engagement with the figure of the cyborg and the informatics of domination: the games of war are messy, and yet in the twenty-first century many of us in the United States are players of one sort or another. To intervene effectively and end the seemingly endless conditions of war making, we must take apart the performed vernaculars that support twenty-first-century state-sponsored violence. To paraphrase Haraway's paraphrase of Gayatri Spivak, to think about our attachments to war is something we cannot afford not to do.[10]

I attempt to address the question of who benefits from war by analyzing specific contexts and fields of material-discursive practices that I hope will be productive of ethical interventions—rather than simplistic disengagements—about what war is doing *for* us now. I qualify in more specific terms how the people in this book are situated in relation to the collective pronouns *we* and *us*, noting how discourses and practices of medical salvation often function to alienate and exclude particular persons and bodies while disavowing this alienation with a language of universal human advancement.

War is now the new everyday. It is striking that the term *postwar* in the United States generally refers to the period after 1945 but is seldom used to describe the periods following the U.S. military occupation of Korea in the 1950s, its withdrawal from Vietnam in the early 1970s, the dissolution of the Soviet Union and hence the Cold War in late 1991, or the nation's participation in the Balkan conflicts of the 1990s. Indeed, as Joseph Masco has argued, the modern national security state apparatus, emerging in 1947, was a product of the long Cold War and has morphed into the Global War on Terror. "The War on Terror," he writes, is "the ideological fulfillment of the Cold War state project, creating an institutional commitment to permanent militarization through an ever-expanding universe of threat identification and response."[11] Focusing on the aim of deterring communism led to the massive expansion of the military-industrial-academic apparatus and to the disciplining of citizens in everyday life. In the years leading up to the suicide-hijacking attacks of September 11, 2001, Americans had been rehearsing the destruction of U.S. cities for over three generations in civil defense drills as well as in watching Hollywood blockbuster movies of the 1990s.[12] By 9/11/01 Americans had been habituated to be ever vigilant. Immediately following the attacks on that day, U.S. officials mobilized the affects of fear, terror, and anger to reconfigure the space and time of military action as unlimited.

We now dwell in an ongoing condition of war at home and abroad against a nebulous enemy called "terror" whose agents are "terrorists." War need no longer be announced by an official declaration for the general population to be in a continual state of attachment to war. It is phrased in a political grammar of xenophobic security against a racialized figure of terror and through which emotional attachment to the state of war permeates myriad affective ways of being. So being "at war" is a constant feeling and a continual state of being that is forged by many quotidian activities and, for the purposes of this book, made manifest in material and biomedical technologies of attachment. The United States and war are themselves inextricably attached to each other in the twenty-first century, as are war and biomedicine. There is no way to be unattached, no such thing as postwar society—unless we begin to intervene in this naturalization and begin to think otherwise.

The idea of attachment in medical and psychological discourses is widely regarded as an enduring emotional bond that normal people have with others. British psychoanalysts developed attachment theory during and following World War II based on observations of infants' various responses to being separated from their primary caregivers. Much of their research was conducted on infants, children, and young adults whose families had been torn apart by war. In controlled clinical studies, researchers found that children who experienced parental psychophysical detachment or indifference tended to exhibit anxiety and fear, whereas those who felt supported were secure, confident, and curious to explore their environment and play with others. Children suffering from prolonged separation experienced profound depression and despair. Described by the psychoanalyst John Bowlby as a motivational system, attachment dynamics were evidenced in infants' crying, clinging, or frantically searching for parents during laboratory-controlled separations out of what Bowlby called a survival technique. The infant, being entirely dependent upon the parent for food and care, expressed demands as a safeguard against extinction until the child was old enough to attend to his or her own needs. Bowlby tied the system to evolutionary pressures of natural selection.[13] Attachment theorists attributed these patterns to the child's sense of loss and helplessness and concluded that strong and supportive emotional bonds between parents and children were necessary for healthy human development into adulthood. They noted too that attachments were relational, not inherent qualities of either the child or the parent, but forged in original as well as ongoing interactions. Though such patterns could also be seen in families not directly affected by it, war was among several key conditions of emotional insecurity dating from infancy and haunting the afflicted into adulthood.

I draw upon this psychological theorizing of attachment but broaden its conceptual field of vision to examine the phenomenological, institutional, and material dimensions of attachment when it comes to the complex affective responses individuals and communities have to notions of defense, security, and belonging. The psychoanalytic model of attachment assumes a normative parent-child dyadic structure. While it does not exclude economic and political factors that may obstruct or negatively affect healthy emotional development, attachment theory tends to focus on the interpersonal dynamics that constitute the well-being or distress of individuals. I extend the concept of attachment in order to consider how ideologies, institutions, expert knowledge, politics, and economic factors attach individuals and a society such as ours to the vast and deep manifestations of militarization that shape our daily realities. These forces and factors paradoxically exploit insecurity as a main motivating condition for authorizing wars. What does it mean for a society to accept that attachment to war is normal? What is offered, promised, or subsumed in this attachment? A complex and contradictory mélange of feelings—many revolving around fear, insecurity, and vengeance but also around hope, caring, and desire for a better future—swirl around in what I refer to as the biomedicine-war nexus. This nexus emerges from a complex set of cultural values and historical developments wherein pervasive and permanent preparedness for war occasions the conditions under which war and biomedicine are bound together in material, affective, ideological, and ethereal ways. War serves biomedicine by producing a steady stream of wounded veterans who become research subjects. National security is imagined as a disease-control surveillance apparatus for detecting deleterious agents, whether persons, pathogens, computer viruses, dangerous attitudes, or toxic assets. In turn, biomedicine serves as a discursive structure and an epistemological tool used by military strategists to draw up battle plans and invade and occupy enemy territory.

Attachments to war manifest in various senses of being and of experiencing life in our thoroughly militarized society. They may manifest as benefits or at least the hope of getting something out of war. Those who stand to profit from it refashion war as a benefit and a necessity to our very lives and bodies. Wounding becomes a boon to the biomedical industry and its shareholders through a political grammar that emphasizes "quality of life" and the "free" pursuit of "health," "longevity," "vitality," "freedom," and other cherished axioms of democracy, all of which are invoked in branding slogans that animate twenty-first-century biomedical war profiteering. Of course war's biomedical and affective benefits are selectively distributed, available to those who can afford them and not to those who are destroyed in war.

Attachments to war manifest in privileging certain types of identity formation and reflect the disciplinary practices that emphasize what it means to be a proper body, a proper citizen, a proper worker, and a proper consumer. Normative "warrior" masculinity, compulsory heterosexuality, nationalist security-motherhood, antiterrorist vigilance, labor flexibility, and willingness to consume the products of militarization—these identification practices divide and categorize who will count as a worthy member of the body politic in whose name the nation's security is invoked. Alongside the behavioral management of war's attachments are its financial entanglements, which may be profitable for some and may manifest in debt and financial ruin for others.

Attachments to war come in the form of a disparate array of promises. Promises at one scale exist in an uneasy relationship to those at another: military recruitment officers are agents of promise when they describe the benefits offered by the GI Bill to high school students in low-income communities where people of color are the majority of residents. These benefits are based on the condition that recruited people are willing to risk their lives. Promises offered to potential investors about the value of shares in biomedical companies are conditioned at least in part on the risks of injury faced by military enlistees. Chances and calculated risks are taken all the time, but for some this is a gamble that could well lead to severe disability or death. It is important to remember that losing share value is not equivalent to losing one's life or health. Anticipating risks and benefits is all part of the deal. In war, some gain fame and fortune, others an existence of unrelenting pain if they manage to survive.

Attachments are often evidenced in the positive emotional conditions of hope, of experiencing a sense of opportunity and of belonging. War galvanizes patriotic cohesion in some people. For some it promises to exact revenge, as Bush pledged following the attacks of 9/11. War now offers enormous economic advantages for weapons manufacturers and their investors as well as for workers employed in war-supported industries. Young enlistees seeking to learn a skill or to get an education in exchange for military service become attached to war as a condition of these promised benefits. War also gives scientists the impetus and the massive funds to undertake world-changing research. To cite a few historical examples, consider the physicists, engineers, and mathematicians who participated in the Manhattan Project to develop the atomic bomb in the latter years of World War II and into the Cold War. Computational scientists funded to conduct Cold War command-control projects produced the knowledge that gave rise to the Internet. During the years surrounding World War II researchers interested in infectious diseases were recruited to the fight against malaria with unprecedented funding. In these large-scale projects scientists were attached to war through their labor. The public was urged to invest great hope in technoscience as a preeminent source of national strength in the context of rapidly escalating geopolitical tensions arising from superpower brinksmanship over who would have control of recently decolonized nations and how extractive and diminishing natural resources would be managed.

Medical science was tied to war at least a century earlier. Modern combat, dating from the Napoleonic wars of the early nineteenth century and the U.S. Civil War of 1861–65, is often credited as the necessary condition under which physicians and scientists made great medical advancements in blood-banking procedures, surgical techniques, pain management, triage measures, and prosthetic rehabilitation. As problematic as this narrative is, it helps to account for the practical ways ordinary people become attached to war as beneficiaries of research funded by militaries and aimed at fighting wars.[14] It has been through the research, development, manufacture, and marketing of pharmaceuticals, implements, and treatments devised in the aftermath of combat to treat its damages that we benefit from war as consumers of these products when they reach the medical market, provided that we have the financial resources to pay for them.

Attachments are relational. They can be strong, fragile, unstable, enduring, motivating, demoralizing, profitable, or devastating. War attaches patients and their loved ones to medical institutions and sets the conditions for what is possible in the way of rehabilitation. Attachments may involve pleasure and hope, but they may also manifest in cathexes to pain, trauma, and dynamics of domination.[15] "A relation of cruel optimism," writes Lauren Berlant, "is a double-bind in which your attachment to an object sustains you in life at the same time as that object is actually a threat to your flourishing."[16] This book explores the apparent contradictions that arise when war is fought in the name of humanity and the resulting bodily devastation is enlisted to recuperate war as a tragic but promising condition. I draw from Berlant the important insight that much can be gained by understanding "how we learn to be in relation" to war—that is, how we are attached to it through what it damages as well as what it promises. Attachments that make up the assemblage entangling biomedicine with war are emotional, political, ideological, and human-technological. Such attachments may hold out hope to the amputee while bringing profit to the prosthetic engineer. They may invest suffering with magical transformational power. They may sunder some relationships in the process of building others; money and investment opportunities come before truly sustained care for the suffering, while loved ones of the damaged lose faith. They may reverberate with the dread of imminent and emergent dangers.

They may reveal that attachments are fragile, as when the nearly destroyed war veteran's patriotic spirit gives way to despair and suicide when the promised rehabilitation fails or never even commences; in 2014 alone, 7,403 veterans killed themselves, a rate of about twenty deaths per day.[17] By 2016 veterans composed 8.5 percent of America's adult population but accounted for 18 percent of its suicides.[18]

Importantly and often, attachments of these sorts are experienced with a deep ambivalence whose symptoms fluctuate among patriotic bellicosity, honorific exaltation, emotional paralysis, and disingenuous disavowal. Some people and institutions benefit from their attachments to war, and others do not. To be attached to war does not necessarily mean to be in support of war. These connections may also manifest in latent symptoms of distress and cognitive dissonance. My point is that these connections are not simply indicative of what a subject or group or society wants or expressly desires; they are, as a matter of some consequence, often haunting reverberations caused by what a subject, group, or society disavows, disregards, or denies. They work to isolate certain persons, bodies, and communities who are cast as blameful targets of enmity or as subjects who are unwilling to comply with something called progress. This book looks at how attachments are generated by a complex matrix of the wounding and sickening capacities of war and at how these capacities haunt the social and psychic lives of sufferers and their sympathizers. It also considers how attachments to war authorize forms of professional prestige and generate speculative portfolios that bring profit to investors enabled by the suffering war causes.

BIOMEDICAL SALVATION

A particularly powerful but largely uninterrogated way that Americans are attached to war is through the complex and hopeful belief that biomedicine offers a salve for violence. The common and enduring account of biomedicine's relationship to war, told across the political spectrum, rehearses a truism that war is horrible and yet it is also an occasion, site, or cause for great innovations and advances of medical knowledge and for devising more humane ways to fight wars. Prominent among the authors of these accounts are journalists who mediate the experience of war in a framework of *biomedical salvation*, a central form of attachment among the many and mixed attachments I analyze.

While lamenting war, purveyors of this narrative note that wars generate large numbers of patients, thus offering opportunities for new knowledge to be gained at a faster rate than from peacetime civilian patient populations whose injuries are staggered across longer durations. As one commenter stated following a National Public Radio report on medical advances at Bagram Airfield in Afghanistan, "These advances would have taken many decades to come about in more peaceful circumstances. The high volume of such catastrophic injuries is why we are getting the opportunity for this research."[19] The flexible ideological configuration of biomedical salvation attaches ordinary citizens to war in a tangled web of sadness, remorse, hope, and gratitude. It also ties biomedicine and war to a volatile economy marked by speculative investments that emphasize futures from a vantage point keen to the opportunities unleashed by an urgent sense of uncertainty, danger, and destruction.

Narratives of biomedical salvation imply that wounds are the necessary precondition for knowledge production. They circulate among medical researchers and physicians who are conducting clinical trials for developing new therapies. They often appear in science-related news stories and on television news features that showcase the wonders of biomedical advances to a targeted audience of educated people nearing or already in retirement. Commercials for vitality-enhancing pharmaceutical products, reverse mortgages, and membership in the AARP offer clues about the intended audience: they are older men and women who recall World War II as a noble triumph over fascism and were steeped in the technoscientific dreams of the Cold War–era space race. Science as secular salvation is a concept to which they are accustomed.

The biomedical salvation narratives of the twenty-first century are in tension with a common sentiment that sees the for-profit health care industry and the military in conflict with one another, particularly over what kind of research receives funding and who is served by the expenditures on these two domains. Antiwar groups see spending on defense as taking funds that could be devoted to health care provision, while hawkish groups argue that "entitlement programs" such as Medicare, Medicaid, and the Affordable Care Act (derisively referred to as "Obamacare") should not take precedence over the nation's military defense. Concerned about whether the Affordable Care Act of 2010 would starve the defense budget while feeding another entitlement program, a columnist writing for the pro-business *Forbes* magazine in 2013 warned that Obamacare would grow so rapidly that federal spending as a share of gross domestic product would increase by more than 40 percent by the year 2085, seriously threatening the nation's defense because it would decrease the amount of money available to spend on armed forces.[20] Biomedical salvation narratives address the conflict between defense spending and entitlement programs through a common media framing that positions biomedical researchers as dedicated to the care of valorized U.S. war-wounded veterans, using the best tools and greatest knowledge available to attend to the suffering of those whose wounds are deemed significant. The knowledge gained by treating these men and women is said to be of value to us all.

A destroy-and-build logic is evident in biomedical salvation narratives and echoes aspects of the U.S.-led military occupations of Afghanistan and Iraq that targeted not only physical infrastructure but also particular bodies for intervention. Creative destruction and the shock doctrine of disaster capitalism infuse this logic.[21] Disaster capitalists take advantage of collective catastrophes. Creative destruction valorizes capitalist innovation as "convulsive," marked by booms and busts. War offers an opportunity to learn things, to come up with new products, to generate profit, or to attract investors with not yet tangible but future life-enhancing things. Wounding and suffering become good for business. Rebuilding is imagined as a chance to radically reshape society and to produce new kinds of citizens who are amenable to free-market capitalism (as entrepreneurs or consumers) and to living in highly militarized occupation zones. It abandons those who are not so amendable.

In the case of biomedical interventions, rehabilitation is akin to rebuilding through its concentration on altering the conditions of future living. In biomedical salvation narratives, war is necessary—dreaded and awful, but necessary—for human advancement. Its destroy-and-build logic exalts the specific nation that goes to war and claims to be an innovator. From at least the last decade of the nineteenth century, when the United States declared war on Spain and extended its imperial reach across the continent and overseas to the east and south, the hegemonic image it has promoted emphasizes industry, commerce, and economic development as expressions of freedom. Bush took the American national brand to a celestial height when he proclaimed, "Americans are a free people, who know that freedom is the right of every person and the future of every nation. The liberty we prize is not America's gift to the world; it is God's gift to humanity. . . . I believe there is an Almighty, and I believe a gift of that Almighty to every man, woman, and child on the face of the Earth is freedom."[22] Enlisting God placed the American empire in a holy valence.

With Bush's placement in the White House in 2001, born-again Christianity had a prominent and vocal spokesperson. His theological orientation was reflected in the terminology he invoked with some frequency when talking about foreign and domestic policy. It was evident, for example, in his intention to wage a "crusade" against "evil-doers" and in his expression of gratitude toward those who were "willing to make the greatest sacrifice" by serving their country in war.[23] Media stories about severely wounded soldiers and marines commonly borrowed elements of this terminology along with biblical precepts emphasized in born-again evangelical Christianity. According to the born-again interpretation of the New Testament, salvation is achieved by God's grace, through which people are delivered from the bondage of sin and condemnation by the sacrifice of Jesus Christ. Christ's atoning sacrifice guarantees eternal life in Heaven for those who have faith—those who have been saved. Christian redemption is generally synonymous with salvation, but its meaning is extended in a secular definition, given by the Oxford English Dictionary, as "the action of regaining or gaining possession of something in exchange for payment, or clearing a debt." To be redeemed can mean either to have atoned for one's errors or sins or, in reference to finance, to clear a debt. Salvation and redemption signify a finite point of resolution. But under the conditions of permanent and pervasive war, they function as ideological mystifications because there is no end point, no Heaven, no possibility of a final repayment of the debt to those who sacrificed. Salvation is unmoored from a terminal point; nor is it eternal. Instead it is ongoing and potentially permanently in play.

Accounts of salvation that tie war to medicine in American popular discourse are certainly not restricted to born-again Christianity. Secular appropriations of salvation are ideologically flexible enough to appeal to a variety of audiences who want to believe that declaring war is honorable when it is done to advance freedom and democracy and when military mobilizations are cast in a benevolent light.[24] Obama's administration, starting in 2008, offset the born-again rhetoric of the Bush administration that preceded him. Obama's pro-science stance against his detractors who doubted the human causes of global climate change and who opposed funding for research using embryonic stem cells put him at considerable distance from Bush. His unofficial renamings of the Global War on Terror to "countering violent extremism" and "overseas contingency operations," together with his rhetorical emphasis on diplomacy and human rights, combined soft and hard power and operated as a strategic principle for authorizing remotely controlled Predator drones as a primary instrument of combat through "targeted assassinations." Salvation narratives transmogrified from their overtly theological quality during the Bush years into a technocratic framing, in which efficiency, precision, and calculated losses came to the fore. Images of returning wounded soldiers all but disappeared from the media, and Obama regularly proclaimed his decision to put "no more boots on the ground." Yet his administration not only increased the number of airborne targeted assassinations but also authorized massive amounts of federal funding for biotechnological research in rehabilitative bionics, regenerative medicine, and biodefense. The funding sutured together public-private partnerships that connected government laboratories to military and veteran administration hospitals, research universities, and biotechnology corporations in a political grammar that combined humane care and forward-looking technoscientific solutions.

Hegemonic accounts of biomedical innovation are subject to modification as presidential administrations change, but even across these differences they continued to resonate with beliefs about salvation. Believers in war-generated biomedicine propped their arguments on a logic of a debt that is owed and that could be repaid but that, under early twenty-first-century finance capitalism, is likely to be projected into a future in which one is urged to speculate in not yet tangible things. Salvation is not a finite or singularly experienced act in this way of thinking about it, but is instead an ongoing process taking place within an assemblage of institutions, disciplinary and market forces, and beliefs. It forms unstable attachments among those planning wars, those fighting wars, those who care for veterans upon their return, those who conduct biomedical research based on veterans' wounds, those who dole out government contracts for research, and those who invest in biomedical stock. Innovations and investments affect people differently depending on contingent conditions such as their access to money and to the cultural resources needed to acquire medical care. Biomedical knowledge and the treatment of wounds caused by war are framed in terms of salvaging the sacrifices made by those who are recognized to bear those wounds, those whose injuries are deemed significant.

Modern war itself is compensated by a notion that war wounds provide the conditions for advancing medical knowledge and aiding humanity. In this secular reframing, war, like sin, is dreadful but also the catalyst for expiation; its wounding capacities generate knowledge and forms of treatment that their creators claim will benefit humanity. The injured or killed body, when recognized as belonging to a significant person (i.e., a patriot or an innocent, not a terrorist or the enemy), is the worthy sacrificial agent; this agent's suffering or death serves to advance biomedical sciences. Biomedical salvation dramatizes American citizens' attachments to the veteran's wounded body as a symbol of sacrifice for which the nation owes a debt. This narrative appears in the chapters that follow.

BIO-INEQUALITY

Throughout the book I pay attention to the unequal evaluations of life that are made visible through the exploitation of biomedicine to justify invasions, security operations, and large expenditures for novel and highly speculative medical treatments. As we will see, much of what is promised for contending with the damage done by war is treatment whose expense is beyond the reach of most people suffering from the consequence of war. The specter of new therapies, devices, and pharmaceutical products casts into the shadows the vast majority of injuries and suffering caused by war today and thus also obscures the means by which they could be ethically addressed. Psychological trauma, illnesses and disabilities caused by exposure to toxic substances, virulent infectious diseases that are resistant to antibiotics, malnutrition, alcoholism and substance abuse, shattered lives—these are among the terrible results of war that manifest in those who are enlisted to fight the wars and in those whom they are fighting to liberate. They are the haunting reality of the biomedicine-war nexus, where miracles do not apply.

Bodies that suffer war wounds are sorted by a variety of social technologies that mark value in relation to distinctions of nationality, race, socioeconomic class, gender, religion, sexuality, and citizenship status. High schools in working-class neighborhoods host military recruiters. Young recruits signify the potential for increasing human capital, as they are trained for specific tasks in the execution of war. Their bodies are worth as much as is invested in their training and in their ability to carry out tasks. If they are injured, their value as human capital is diminished or terminated.

The U.S. Army gives away video games to teenage boys and young men in working-class communities where other job opportunities are absent or, at best, limited. It promises immigrants an accelerated path to citizenship for enlisting. It hails men and women who want to go to college but cannot pay the tuition. It targets athletes and sports fans through mass advertising during the Super Bowl and the NBA Finals and in previews of action adventure movies. It sends "grunts" and "cannon fodder"—low-ranking men and women from humble origins—into the line of fire. It offers pay bonuses for those willing and eligible for combat. If they are wounded in action, they are promised care and rehabilitation and monetary compensation, but the delivery falls far short of the promise and the cost to taxpayers is overwhelming.[25]

Material realities offset the benefits promised by the military and by biomedicine, providing evidence of how certain lives are valued over others. The first concerns the biomedical industry's development of high-tech, expensive, and lifelong therapies that are too costly for the vast majority of persons wounded in war—besides U.S. troops, the many whose lands were invaded, their communities destroyed, and their bodies devastated by battle. With the costs of medical insurance and treatment rapidly rising, even basic care is too expensive for many wounded U.S. service members. Bureaucratic inefficiencies in medical record keeping, a shortage of physicians and other medical personnel, and a backlog of compensation claims vastly impede care for many returning veterans.[26] This, coupled with the contraction of social welfare benefits, results in increasing rates of poverty and unemployment among wounded U.S. veterans, particularly among the enlisted ranks, where men and women of color are concentrated.[27]

Bio-inequality—the outcome of procedures that value some lives over others—is partly a product of social determinants of health.[28] These are factors that either promote or endanger an individual or a community's health and vitality. Communities that enjoy better housing, schools, and medical care and higher incomes generally enjoy greater health. Stressful working conditions, decrepit living conditions, poverty, unemployment, violence, lack of access to healthy food, air, and water, lack of educational opportunities, lack of access to medical care, and the ready availability of illicit drugs and alcohol put impoverished communities at risk for higher rates of infant mortality and chronic disease as well as shorter life expectancy. No magic therapy, sensational pharmaceutical, or miracle device can make up for the health-endangering effects of poverty and failing public services and medical infrastructure. Yet many of the returning U.S. veterans from wars fought in Iraq and Afghanistan came from (and go back to) communities with poor social determinants of health and, while a select few are offered novel therapies, most lack the resources to contend with endemic social factors that endanger their health.

There is a tension here about the status of the veteran: in many ways service members—especially those occupying the lower ranks—are routinely subjected to harm and then neglected by the Veterans Administration's inadequacies. But it could be argued that veterans (at least those who manage to breach the threshold of access to meaningful VA services) are a privileged group. The system to which they have access is periodically under intense scrutiny for political reasons, and therefore seems to be irreparably broken every few years or so, but it is arguably quite functional relative to the paucity of options available to others.

The situation is much worse for wounded Iraqi and Afghan citizens, the vast majority of whom have had little or no access to medical care after the U.S. invasion of their communities. Resource extraction and establishing new horizons for financial speculation were central to the logics and practices of waging war in Afghanistan and Iraq. And in many ways these practices intentionally endangered the lives and livelihoods of those who were being "saved from tyranny." Recall, for example, that the Bush administration launched the Global War on Terror in the name of humanity to rid the world of "evil-doers" and to bring freedom to those living under tyrannical rule in the "Axis of Evil."[29] This declaration resulted in nearly half a million war-generated deaths of Iraqi citizens and a conservative estimate of between 12,500 and 14,700 Afghan civilians from 2001 to 2011. A comprehensive study of war- and occupation-related deaths among soldiers and civilians in Iraq between 2003 and 2011 determined that "beyond expected rates, most mortality increases in Iraq [from previous studies] can be attributed to direct violence, but about a third are attributable to indirect causes (such as from failures of health, sanitation, transportation, communication, and other systems). Approximately a half million deaths in Iraq could be attributable to the war."[30] The figures for war-related deaths in Afghanistan were less rigorously recorded, but an estimate of between 30,400 and 45,600 (including civilians, Afghan military, police, insurgents, aid workers, and journalists) died due to the war there between October 2001 and June 2011.[31]

In addition to these deaths, Bush's declaration manifested in establishing laws friendly to privately held corporations for "rebuilding" Iraq and Afghanistan that undermined the health and nutrition of local populations.

A notable example is the outlawing in 2002 of heirloom seeds in Iraq by L. Paul Bremer, Bush's appointee to head the Coalition Provisional Authority following the fall of Saddam Hussein's regime. The new law governing intellectual property required that Iraqi farmers abandon a practice they had been using for centuries and instead obtain a yearly license to repurchase seeds from an authorized supplier, or face a fine or penalty.[32] Comply or starve: these were the options. Bush declared war in the name of remaking Iraqi society in the mode of free-market capitalism and, if not only for oil, for a long list of natural resources and speculative investment opportunities tangled up in the ever-expanding market for biotechnology, surveillance, and security, at home and abroad. Certain bodies were marked for care, and others, if not killed, were mistreated or abandoned to die. Within a year of the U.S.-led invasion of Iraq, half of the country's 26 million people were unemployed or underemployed; 400,000 of these were soldiers who lost their positions when Bremer abolished the invaded nation's army. During this period the homes of Iraqi citizens were routinely raided by U.S. troops. Many men were arrested and detained indefinitely, subject to harsh interrogation and torture. Within the first six months after the invasion, an estimated 7,900 to 9,800 Iraqi civilians died due to war-related causes. The U.S. military's procedure for compensating civilian deaths was secretive, inconsistent, and shamefully modest, with a discretionary $2,500 "condolence payment" for civilian deaths for which the United States offered "an expression of sympathy" but "without reference to fault."[33] Compensation payments for deaths varied widely but seldom exceeded $5,000. Compensation for children's deaths was generally no greater than for adults, despite the normative calculations of human capital used by the World Bank that estimates the statistical value of life in the United States between $3 million and $5 million. Educated young adults, according to this calculation, are worth more than children who have not yet acquired skills and are worth more than older adults, especially the elderly, who have fewer years of income earning left.[34]

We see in these developments an economization of life in which there is a biopolitical equation: some must die so that others may live. This is an equation that follows a lineage from twentieth-century eugenics movements to modern genocides of that century to development-based population control campaigns and now to macroeconomic cost-benefit calculations of the value of human capital, according to which, as Michelle Murphy has noted, some must die or be abandoned for the sake of the aggregate population and its improvement.[35] Overt racialization, in these more recent technocratic discourses, is submerged beneath a language of cost-effective investment about who will lead a productive life (i.e., who will enhance the gross domestic product of a nation and contribute to its economy or to its debt repayment to the IMF). The reproductive politics of IMF and World Bank macroeconomic policy in the twenty-first century sort those, on the one hand, who are deemed worthy of education and who promise future productivity from, on the other hand, those who are disposable and whose lives are even preventable. As Murphy writes, "Some must not be born so that future others will live more abundantly, consumptively, productively."[36] Bodies and lives of war-damaged Afghan and Iraqi people do not populate the hegemonic narrative of biomedical salvation. Instead they join the massive surplus population of the twenty-first century of many millions of people who, because of catastrophic displacement caused by imperial ventures to seize resources, can no longer eke out a living. They exist, as Aaron Benanav and John Clegg explain, "only to be managed: segregated into prisons, marginalized in ghettos and camps, disciplined by the police, or annihilated by war."[37]

CHAPTER OUTLINES

The attachments that animate this book are, centrally, those of ordinary American citizens to war, which is itself forged through attachments to biomedicine, understood as both a tangible industry and a set of promising fantasies. These are tied to political ideologies and affective phenomena that, together, create a biomedicine-war nexus that is centered on the notion of care, the focus of chapter 1. The biomedicine-war nexus produces new subdisciplines and novel war-generated diagnoses and rehabilitative innovations, as I detail in chapter 2, drawing the American hero or martyr (troops) into intimacy with teams of biomedical specialists represented as miracle workers in media stories about them. Audiences are positioned through these narratives to mourn the extreme damages done by war and to honor the bodies of wounded martyrs by beholding the experimental genius of rehabilitation and regeneration from the new medically codified diagnosis of *polytrauma*. This is one of several key ways that technoscientific and biomedical promises provide a means through which attachments to war persist. Military physicians classify polytrauma as a "signature injury." As such, in my analysis, the devastating phenomenon indexes a particular kind of *woundscape* and requires special reading practices to interpret the significance that is attributed to the injury both in biomedical and political terms.[38] The woundscapes of significantly injured patients—American troops—prompt an indebtedness whereby the nation owes twice for the sacrifices made: once for the wound acquired as the warrior served the nation and again for the new knowledge that can be derived from medical treatment of the warrior's suffering. Bodies of those whose injuries do not rise to the level of significance—those who are among the surplus or disposable population—are symptomatically missing from the biomedical salvation tales of polytrauma treatment.

Chapter 3, on bionic innovations, is concerned with the phenomenon of *biomedicalization* as it opens the door for future investments in the biomedicine-war nexus. Biomedicalization is a forward-looking convergence that is enabled by advancements in molecular biology, biotechnology, transplant and regenerative medicine, and genomics.[39] It emphasizes transformations of medical phenomena in interventions aimed not simply at curing or treating the body but at enhancing or augmenting its functions. Medical intervention for the sake of improvement becomes normalized. Think, for instance, of pills to augment erectile function, preemptive mastectomies for preventing cancer, and drugs to enhance cognitive concentration and memory. Think too about how it is now possible to survive complete heart failure, to give birth decades after menopause, to walk without leg bones, and to genetically design life. The promises of military medicine often turn on claims for the potential of war-generated medical treatments to enhance, augment, and transform every body's abilities.

In chapter 3 I trace how the biomedicine-war nexus manufactures knowledge that materializes in biomedical devices that are literally attachments, as in the case of bionic prosthetics—devices to which we attach major emotional, political, and health significance. Paradoxically the bodies of severely wounded veterans of recent wars—those who, under previous conditions, would not have survived—are figured centrally in narratives of the future enhancement and the expanded potential of human bodies. Their injuries afford the inventors of bionic prosthetics opportunities to demonstrate the promise of technoscientific innovations. The carefully crafted performances of bodily augmentation are presented to audiences who, often unwittingly, became further attached to war through what bioengineering promises not only for injured veterans but for everyone. By witnessing what can be done to restore amputees' otherwise lost abilities, audiences are invited to look forward to a future when bioengineering may enable humanity to go beyond a host of bodily limitations.

Chapter 4 focuses on pathogens used in war and confronts a situation in which the bodies of soldiers are not ultimately exceptional. Instead, in the face of imminent and emergent pathogens, all bodies are conceived as potentially threatened or threatening, and some more threatening than others. Ordinary people become attached to war through a terrified sense of being quietly and covertly attacked at the micro level by new and more virulent mutating germs, viruses, and toxins, whether by intentional acts or accidental exposure. Bodies are in this sense potentially both targets and weapons—victims and vectors—in the apocalyptic framing of ominous doom. War is waged on, through, and with microscopic pathogens. Panic is a marketing tool. Fear is an investment stimulator for biotechnology companies developing products to detect, treat, and contain imminent and predicted biological threats. Counterterror biotechnical strategies are speculative in two main ways: seeing into the future is a central dynamic of the emerging global health apparatus, where threat detection and risk assessment have taken on apocalyptic proportions. Making bets on what products may be most effective in containing and countering emergent pathogenic agents involves financial speculation on not yet existing but absolutely necessary biotechnology. There is no territorial or temporal limit to the new bio-imperialism emanating out of the U.S. state's investment in securing life against biological threats. Life must be secured on a global scale in the name of domestic defense, a planetary project driven by fearful intuitions and end-of-the-world scenarios.

ONE

The Biomedicine-War Nexus

National security, warfare, and biomedical logics form a nexus in which deliberate violence—war—is bound up with far-reaching aspirations about improving life. Biomedical logics associate medicine with an ethic of care. As such, when they are mobilized in domestic policing or in imperial military operations, they function to obscure the causes and effects of violence. This obfuscation accounts for some of the ways attachments to war manifest: an affective investment in care resides at the heart of the biomedicine-war nexus. Discourses of care authorize security measures that divide the beneficial from the deleterious, the healthy from the pathological, and those who deserve security from those who threaten it, at home and in overseas military interventions.

Biomedical logics form part of the nation's arsenal and an integral part of its surveillance apparatus, organized around the tropes of defense and security. They gain considerable momentum when fear, dread, and xenophobic paranoia expand the militarization of everyday life in the name of homeland security. They operate in allegorical renderings in which warfare and mechanisms aimed at ensuring national security are conceived as medical operations. Within these allegories biomedical logics serve as epistemological tools—devices for thinking—used by military strategists to draw up battle plans and to carry out counterinsurgency operations in imperial occupations. They play an important role in the destroy-and-build dynamics through which new disciplinary regimes are imposed upon occupied communities. Military strategists exploit medicine's ethic of care to carry out covert operations that actually undermine the health and security of the very people the operations are claiming to liberate. Biomedical logics rationalize violence and, through their association with an ethic of care, attach people to war.

This chapter begins with a contextualizing account of the militarization of everyday life, arguing that ordinary citizens are attached to war through the mobilization of fear and insecurity. I then examine the various ways that biomedicine has become militarized, particularly in the context of U.S. military operations in Afghanistan and Iraq. I review specific biomedical practices that were deployed as instruments of violence and show how clinics were transformed into strategic targets. Militarized biomedicine not only encompasses the enlistment of medical professionals to carry out violence but also manifests in an insidious violence that is couched in military counterinsurgency doctrine that purports to care for compliant inhabitants of occupied regions.

A discursive analysis of counterinsurgency doctrine reveals how the violence of war is obscured and sanitized by metaphors and allegories likening battle and occupation to urgent medical interventions. The invading and occupying force is staged metaphorically as an expert medical team whose main task is to rid the occupied society of a diseased insurgency, transforming the ill patient into a compliant subject of the new occupying regime. Women and children in the occupied regions are the focus of rescue campaigns that seize upon the promise of health care to draw them into counterinsurgency plans. A deadly consequence is that medical facilities become targets of insurgent attacks. Postinvasion policies that radically transformed life in Afghanistan and Iraq focused on eliminating socialized medicine and introducing privatized medical care. Clinics and hospitals were strategic targets exploited not only in counterinsurgency operations but also in neoliberal economic policies that destroyed the existing health care systems and did little to address the catastrophic outcome of this destruction. In the name of care, the occupying forces did much to endanger the lives of the occupied, whose trust in the medical profession eroded substantially as corruption and covert operations threw their communities into chaos.

In the final section I reflect on bio-equality, noting that a politics of life is closely linked with a politics of death in a discursive circuitry whereby some lives are honored as worthy sacrificial heroes while others are calculated to be expendable. An economy of life according to which some bodies are valued and others are disposable underlies a particular kind of attachment to war, one centered on advancement and grounded deeply in a faith and devotion to technological innovation that claims to be humane and thus justifies violence as a necessary condition for human advancement.

MILITARIZATION OF EVERYDAY LIFE: THE HOMELAND

Americans are attached to war through the militarization of everyday life in which the elements that are constitutive of war—enmity, exclusion, existential threat, emergency, the foregrounding of distinctions between "us" and "them," policing tactics, surveillance, and violence—permeate social and political relationships. I define *militarization* as an ongoing process aimed at the management and disciplining of populations staged in the name of defending society. Combatants are ubiquitous and include not only dangerous people but also biological and computer viruses, toxic assets, virulent proteins, bad attitudes, malfunctioning systems, political dissent, and faulty intelligence information. All around us we hear the message "Be afraid. Be very, very afraid." Tactics of population management are embedded in our institutions, constitutive of who we are, embodied in our physical comportment, performed in our daily lives, and exported to other regions through new modes of colonialism. War tactics and technologies are commanding expectations down to bodies as sites of imposing order through discipline and regulation. We are compelled to police ourselves by being encouraged to police Others, in the name of security. Militarization colonizes minds and bodies as well as spaces near and far.

The University of Chicago sociologist Robert E. Park anticipated this condition of permanent and pervasive war when he wrote that "psychic warfare" was a central feature of what he called *total war* societies. Published in the *American Journal of Sociology* in November 1941, just a month before President Franklin Delano Roosevelt declared war on Japan and Germany, Park endorsed a vigilant state of psychological preparedness as a necessary dimension of war: "Total war is now an enterprise so colossal that belligerent nations find it necessary not only to mobilize all their resources, material and moral, but also to make present peace little more than a preparation for future war."[1]

Total war society became a term of art for describing the necessary conditions for ensuring modern national defense, a concept used by mid-twentieth-century military and civilian war strategists but with roots dating back to the establishment of mass-conscripted armies in new European nation-states in the late eighteenth century. It is a formation of modern industrialized states with colonies and empires. Total war, thus conceived, is a circumstance in which all significant sectors of society are mobilized for the purposes of defending a nation. Vannevar Bush, Roosevelt's director of the Office of Scientific Research and Development, writing at the end of World War II, quoted a joint letter sent to the National Academy of Sciences by the Secretaries of War and the Navy: "This war emphasizes three facts of supreme importance to national security: (1) powerful new tactics of defense and offense are developed around new weapons created by scientific and engineering research; (2) the competitive time element in developing those weapons and tactics may be decisive; (3) war is increasingly *total war*, in which the armed services must be supplemented by active participation of every element of civilian population."[2]

In total war society, industrial, agricultural, communications, and transportation systems are geared toward the effort. Scientific, medical, technical, and other professional talent is drawn into the duty to defend the nation and support its military. Schools, colleges, laboratories, and media assume important roles in war preparedness. Civil society, religious institutions, and the industry of mass media are absorbed into the venture. Total war is total mobilization and total preparedness. It requires extensive centralized planning and control while also scattering hegemony through distributed circuits of enforcement. It necessitates popular compliance or the means to effectively quell popular dissent. Preparedness and the constant productions it requires in industry, finance, politics, and ideology exist prior to the formal declaration of war and persist past the official pronouncement of a war's conclusion.

Total war's institutional moorings and the economic investments that support it become endemic to the society. Demilitarization is unthinkable because so many industries rely on total war for profit and political influence and because the nation's security is ideologically premised on having a highly armed state. This was one of Dwight D. Eisenhower's concerns, when in 1960 he delivered the last public address of his presidency, warning against "the acquisition of unwarranted influence, whether sought or unsought, by the military-industrial complex." But Eisenhower, speaking in the context of the Cold War, regarded it as necessary that the United States have a "permanent armaments industry of vast proportion" to defend against "a hostile ideology—global in scope, atheistic in character, ruthless in purpose, and insidious in method. . . . This conjunction of an immense military establishment is new in the American experience. The total influence—economic, political, and even spiritual—is felt in every city, every Statehouse, every office of the Federal government. We recognize the imperative need for this development. Yet we must not fail to comprehend its grave implications. Our toil, resources and livelihood are all involved; *so is the very structure of our society.*"[3]

Total war blurs the boundaries between the soldier and the civilian, between security operations and military operations, between the home and the combat zone, between war and peace, and between affective dispositions and military tactics. As Jackie Orr has argued, total war officially drafts the U.S. civilian into being a military combatant who is expected to take an active psychological role in the conduct of successful war.[4] The concept of a total war society further materialized in the vigilance of emergency drills during the Cold War between the Soviet Union and the United States, when mutually assured destruction (MAD) was the doctrine through which popular images of world-eviscerating weapons propelled the building of home bomb shelters, the stockpiling of guns and supplies, and suspicion that one's coworkers and neighbors might be spies for the enemy. The specter of nuclear war taught ordinary citizens to incorporate a sense of living constantly under the existential threat of potential obliteration. In this zero-sum game, citizens were compelled to learn how to defend the nation against an apocalyptic fate and to accept nuclear detonation tests, stockpiling of weapons of mass destruction, and civil defense drills as necessary and quotidian aspects of life. Discourses of ruination were integral to U.S. nation-building in the age of atomic warfare. The theater of operations was planetary in reach and the time of war indefinite in duration.[5]

By the advent of the Global War on Terror, our total war society had become networked by cybernetic circuits of information technology that cross platforms of war planning, border control, logistics management, financial transactions, media entertainments, and biomedical research. The nation had developed and stockpiled massive weapons systems, implemented a widespread apparatus of surveillance, built scores of laboratories dedicated to research on biodefense and biosecurity, established clinics and hospitals to contain deadly infectious pathogens and the bodies that contain them, and funded university research centers dedicated to projects of prediction and the logistics of security and warfare. Following the suicide and hijacking attacks of 9/11, this far-flung national security apparatus expanded massively, ideologically fulfilling the Cold War state project, creating, as Joseph Masco notes, "an institutional commitment to permanent militarization though an ever-expanding universe of threat and detection."[6]

Security has become a central engine of the economy and an opportunity for employment, profiteering, and financial speculation. Private enterprises pitch product ideas to government agencies, seeking to secure grants and contracts to manufacture stuff that claims to be of service to national security—bombs, vaccines, bullets, surveillance devices, simulation software, prosthetic limbs, business models, to name just a few. Identifying threats is a focus of myriad branches of the state as well as of private enterprises where surveillance, profiling, and targeting reflect a logic that is internalized in individuals as well as built into a diffuse apparatus, or what Foucault called a "disciplinary corpus."[7] Prisons and detention centers proliferate. Guard labor becomes a growing sector of employment.[8] For-profit detention centers extract wealth from the disposable life of "illegals." Technologies of surveillance are packaged into consumer-grade commodities and incorporate acts of spying into daily life routines through mobile phones, global positioning systems, and biomonitoring devices.[9] Hospitals and medical clinics become guarded locations where patients must show proper identification and pass through metal detectors and other surveillance screenings and where armed employees are stationed to apprehend undocumented people or anyone warranting suspicion. In the name of national security, the health of Others is severely compromised.

Meanwhile threats and dangers are also summoned as beneficial. In Bush's 2002 State of the Union address to Congress, he promised that his proposed expansion of homeland security measures would do more than simply stave off enemies: "Homeland security will make America not only stronger, but, in many ways, better. Knowledge gained from bioterrorism research will improve public health. Stronger police and fire departments will mean safer neighborhoods. Stricter border enforcement will help combat illegal drugs. And as government works to better secure our homeland, America will continue to depend on the eyes and ears of alert citizens."[10] These new efforts deepened the public's attachments to war in the political grammar of security. Bush tied the geopolitics of border control to the biopolitics of combating illegal drugs. "Alert citizens" were enlisted as unpaid guard labor. And an apocalyptic orientation toward the future coexisted with a promise of being saved by incorporating and putting into routine performance the embedded knowledges developed in the name of security.[11]

Alert citizens enjoy a kind of vigilant sovereignty with which they are encouraged to patrol and apprehend suspicious characters and take violent action against them if necessary, often governed by a disavowed racist logic that validates the targeting of people of color in the United States.[12] The phenomenon was dramatized in the acquittal of George Zimmerman for killing an unarmed seventeen-year-old African American, Trayvon Martin, who was visiting his father in a condominium complex in February 2012. In his defense Zimmerman invoked the state of Florida's "stand your ground" law, which permits citizens to use violent force against intruders or anyone who appears to threaten the citizen's safety. A Florida jury acquitted Zimmerman, who never denied shooting Martin, of second-degree murder and manslaughter charges in the summer of 2013.

The alert citizen is hailed in the "If you see something, say something™" campaign sponsored by the U.S. Department of Homeland Security and originally developed by the Metropolitan Transportation Authority in New York City. The campaign's slogan captures this sentiment in its claim of being "a simple and effective program to engage the public and key frontline employees to identify and report indicators of terrorism and terrorism-related crime to the proper transportation and law authorities."[13] Alert citizens are encouraged to tell the proper authorities about suspicious activity. Within a larger context in which racial profiling is endemic to official policing actions and citizens are warned of the dangerous presence of "loitering youth" and the potential dangers posed by people of Middle Eastern descent or those assumed to be Muslim, suspicious activities can include standing with friends on the street in front of one's home, praying on an airplane, walking or driving in certain parts of town, wearing certain kinds of clothing (head scarves or turbans or hooded sweatshirts, for example), and speaking in certain kinds of accented English.

America's security apparatus also conditions access to employment, housing, medical care, and education. Biomedical procedures are integral to screening people for eligibility or disqualification. Private employers mandate drug testing and background checks of potential employees, again in the name of securing the enterprise against risks and threats. Recipients of public assistance are required to submit to drug tests. Health insurance companies require that individuals report previous medical problems—"preexisting conditions"—so that the companies may minimize their economic risk by excluding those with such conditions or charging them more for coverage. We are prompted to be self-monitoring and self-regulating for the sake of minimizing risk. Watch your weight, stop smoking, and take only the drugs your doctor has prescribed.

National security is also framed as a medical problem, manifesting in the fear of pandemics, biological weapons of mass destruction, and bioterrorism.[14] Biomedical logics increasingly infuse the world of security policy, placing medical and health professionals centrally in the process of tracking and containing outbreaks and isolating "threat vectors." Medical countermeasures are produced and stockpiled in preparation for potential viral outbreaks. Security extends to a focus on the inner workings of the human organism, where citizens and military personnel are transformed into patients by mandated vaccinations or compulsory quarantine in anticipation of disease outbreaks. Biomedical procedures are brought into the prosecution of war, as, for example, in the development of performance-enhancing drugs for maximizing troop activities in combat, as well as the enforcement of biosecurity through mandated ingestion of pharmaceutical prophylaxes.

Biomedicine becomes a vector through which people are to perform the duty to be healthy, to seek out appropriate medical treatment when needed, and to be low risk, even if they lack the financial means or access to health care to fulfill these duties. In other words, operating within an increasingly securitized society characterized by the polarization of wealth and poverty and racialized social dispossession, biomedicine becomes a vehicle for tacitly reducing some people to disposable life, a process that is obscured by the rhetoric of technological triumphalism that supports increasingly expensive and speculative biomedical futures available only to the few who can afford them. Biomedical logics, marshaled to the nation's security, extend beyond its territorial borders to rationalize violent invasions and imperial occupations as preemptive operations.

MILITARIZED BIOMEDICINE: THE OCCUPIED REGIONS

Biomedicine is militarized in several key ways in the context of the twenty-first-century U.S. military occupation of Afghanistan and Iraq. First is the *practical deployment* of medical procedures as instruments of war by withholding care from anyone labeled a terrorist, criminalizing medical personnel who provide care to enemies, overseeing the force-feeding of detainees waging hunger strikes, and using medical knowledge and instruments to inflict torture or to gather biometric information from invaded populations.[15] Second, biomedicine is militarized through the use of medical metaphors for describing various kinds of combat operations, which function to sanitize or euphemize acts of violence and their effects. Configuring the enemy as inherently diseased, degenerate, and infectious is an ideological habit that manifested in many varieties of colonial ventures of Western modernity.[16] This habit persists in postmodern military operations but with important shifts, most notably in the prominence of technocratic humanitarian reasoning that is used for rationalizing particular strategies of intervention and occupation. Though the Bush administration's neoconservative expansionism differed substantially from the "smart power" of Obama's humanitarian interventionism, both approaches made claims for legitimacy on the grounds of caring for ordinary people living under despotic regimes.[17] The Bush administration favored military occupation and nation-building, while Obama preferred carrot-and-stick diplomacy and, when deemed necessary, special operations and drone strikes.

Perhaps the most common among the medical metaphors of this technocratic humanitarianism is the "surgical strike," a commonplace to describe purported precision in targeted bombing and a necessary and urgent operation akin to removing a tumor or other deleterious agent through a penetrating incision and extraction carried out by a skilled expert with the appropriate technological devices. "Collateral damage" is analogous to the side effect of a necessary medical treatment: according to this logic, the deaths and injuries of ordinary noncombatant people harmed inadvertently by precision targeting are regrettable but also the result of the necessary risks taken. The metaphorical traffic moves back and forth between medicine and war, deepening the signification apparatus they share. Think, for example, of the allegorical war on cancer, in which a medical team wages a battle, with the ailing patient's cooperation, to destroy cancerous tissue by means of chemotherapy or by surgical intervention.

The metaphor of a war waged against disease puts patients in the role of warriors. The patient's friends, families, and communities are engaged in the combat as supportive foot soldiers. Worthy combatants and their allies in the fight have available to them a proliferating wardrobe of awareness ribbons to indicate their commitment to do battle: pink for the war on breast cancer and yellow for the war on terror. Physicians are cast as the commanders drawing up and executing the battle plans. The medicine that is administered is intentionally lethal, targeted at killing the cancer cells but routinely giving rise to collateral effects that belong to that family of medical problems known as iatrogenic ailments caused by the medical treatment itself. Dosage levels are indexed to an economy of life in which the cancer cell is killed for the sake of regenerating the life of the patient.

Counterinsurgency Operations as Medical Interventions

A third manifestation of militarized biomedicine appears in military doctrine and strategic planning. Counterinsurgency operations (or COIN operations, their official acronym) are imagined in what Colleen Bell has insightfully called "the allegory of medical intervention."[18] Authors of counterinsurgency doctrine emphasized the population-centric qualities of this kind of military intervention, distinguishing it from an enemy-centric framework of combat warfare. The doctrine's controversial human terrain systems program used military personnel and private contractors trained in social and behavioral sciences to conduct sociocultural research on occupied populations in order to support and enhance operational effectiveness.[19]

Though the counterinsurgency doctrine claims to be population-centric, Bell notes that it produces a kind of hybrid warfare, one that "articulates a politics of life and regeneration, amid the death and destruction that accompanies war."[20] It simultaneously enacts targeted killing while compelling the population to live, employing overtly coercive and putatively noncoercive tactics toward the goal of eradicating insurgency. The emphasis in COIN operations is on what its proponents call cultural awareness and effective communication with an occupied population. These campaigns propose security operations and humanitarian interventions to win the hearts and minds of the population of the host nation. They aim to marginalize and ultimately exterminate insurgent tactics, ideas, and people. The allegory of medical intervention reflects the kind of warfare that technocratic proponents of counterinsurgency *wish* it to be, despite repeated evidence that COIN operations play out in messy ways that defy military doctrine.

According to the medical allegory's principles, the key characters in the story are the physician, the illness, and the patient. As Bell observes, this casting of characters allows the counterinsurgents to be positioned as benevolent experts, while the insurgents are portrayed as destructive and alien. The population is, like a patient, the battleground (or "human terrain") of the conflict. Bell writes, "The allegory draws on the authority and perceived objectivity of medicine to produce a charitable understanding of the purpose and function of counterinsurgency warfare." And the allegorical structure, she observes, is not simply a guide to operations but also "a self-serving, political campaign to improve the morale of weary soldiers and soothe anxious publics in the midst of war."[21]

The U.S. Army and Marine Corps's *Counterinsurgency: Field Manual 3-24*, released in December 2006, embodies the allegorical structure of medical intervention by describing counterinsurgency as a therapeutic operation that follows what the authors refer to as three "indistinct" stages.[22] At each stage the goal is to gain the cooperation of the patient in order to acquire useful information that can lead to the defeat of insurgent forces. In the initial stage its experts must "stop the bleeding" caused by a contagion stage, wherein insurgent ideas, like an influenza virus, "bleed out" into the population that is already suffering from a weakened immune system. Experts perform emergency "first aid" on the patient or population to stop the bleeding. The aim is to "shap[e] the information environment" as a way to contain the deleterious influence of insurgents. Such procedures may include educational campaigns, development programs, and the offer to provide actual health care, but all are enforced by the presence of armed forces. Next the experts conduct "inpatient care—recovery" in order to stabilize the population and place it on a path toward "restoration of health," defined as achieving compliance and stability. A key element in this process is strengthening the "flow of human and other types of intelligence," which "facilitates measured offensive operations" and works toward the goal of increasing the legitimacy of the host nation (for example, the Islamic Republic of Afghanistan, established under the aegis of the U.S.-led coalition in 2004) by "providing essential services." Finally, in the "late stage," the patient is released to "outpatient" care, in which the population is enabled to move toward self-sufficiency and stability.[23]

Throughout the allegory insurgents have no social identities but are merely disease agents or "festering elements" in the patient's body, threatening to spread if an intervention is not performed. The tripartite process of *clear-hold-build* that military strategists refer to as the summation of a successful military occupation is transmuted in the counterinsurgency allegory into *quarantine–risk reduction–behavioral modification*. The disease of insurgency is defeated by healing interventions that use "soft-and-smart power" (i.e., humanitarian, reconstructive, and diplomatic methods) to protect and strengthen the body. Eventually the body, as an allegorical figure for the new regime, will ideally gain the ability to take over its own security operations and be less dependent on foreign assistance (i.e., U.S.

or NATO forces). The *Field Manual* warns that coercive measures should be used with great care and sparingly by targeting the cause of the disease (the insurgent) in order to minimize the suffering of the patient (the population) so that he or she does not become alienated and disinvested in the healing process.

David Kilcullen, a principal author of counterinsurgency doctrine, extended the allegory further into the terrain of immunology. As commander of the Multi-National Forces in Iraq, U.S. Army General David Petraeus applied Kilcullen's ideas in the troop surges conducted in Iraq in 2007 and later in Afghanistan in 2009. The ultimate goal of counterinsurgency, Kilcullen declared, is to restore the population's immune system following an alien infection. In other words, counterinsurgency is a way to help a population reject foreign elements that threaten its health. He warned that the population may have an initial "autoimmune rejection" of the assistance provided by intervention. Like the body's rejection of a "pin in a broken bone or a stent in a blocked blood vessel," the population may attack the beneficial agent (i.e., the doctrine of COIN operations as well as the troops charged with implementing it) rather than attacking the real "foreigner," the insurgent. Following this reasoning and through a hubristic sleight of hand, the actual foreign invader—the U.S.-led coalition forces in Iraq and Afghanistan—is replaced by a new foreigner: the insurgent who opposes the intended order of occupation and is foreign to the host nation's new authority. Ultimately Kilcullen advised that the population should be "inoculated" against the insurgency in order to direct its immune system toward advancing counterinsurgency goals of stabilization and self-sufficiency for the host nation. The goal of this whole therapeutic exercise is to fortify the new regime's self-defense capabilities through such activities as recruiting and training new police forces and national armies who will eventually be able to assume the security operations in the region and contain or exterminate the insurgency. If the population rejects these training opportunities or various kinds of aid, the counterinsurgency operation has failed. To ensure against this undesired outcome, counterinsurgency "demands the continuous presence of security forces," "local alliances and partnerships with community leaders that operate in tandem with local security forces."[24] It is likely, in other words, to require the long-term presence of armed enforcement agents carrying out the interests of the beneficial agent, particularly if the patient is noncomplying. Occupation is, in a sense, a chronic condition that requires ongoing therapeutic attention.

Casting counterinsurgency as a therapeutic process mystifies the brutality and indiscriminate violence carried out against civilians in the name of a larger regenerative process. If the patient is uncooperative, it is the therapist or physician who must make the patient comply for his or her own good. "Supporting, or acquiescing to, the insurgency is figured as a consequence of being sick," writes Bell. "Health, therefore, stands in for correct desires."[25] The allegory of medical intervention, like all allegories, tells a story for the sake of presenting a truth. Its primary audience is military strategists who acknowledge that wars cannot be won simply with high-tech weapons and scorched-earth tactics. But it also tells this story to the U.S. tax-paying public that pays for military operations around the world and is urged to find comfort in thinking that these operations are actually forms of benevolence and care. The targeted population, whose support counterinsurgency operatives seek, is a much less significant audience for the tale. The allegory—like counterinsurgency doctrine itself—exists mainly in the realm of fantasy. Given that insurgents in Iraq were not foreign to the population, and given that the therapeutic claims of COIN operations were defied by the violence and insecurity that they unleashed, the allegory broke down in practice. A war-weary U.S. public became disillusioned or, worse, resentful, while people living under military occupation had good reason to doubt that the therapy they were being administered was any better than the disease. Despite its failure, the allegory of intervention as caring, efficient, and medicinal persisted throughout the Obama years, indicating its durable appeal for rationalizing violence through a biomedical valence.

Rescue Narratives: Gender Strategies of Counterinsurgency Operations

In the history of colonialism and in the present, counterinsurgency is a gendered formation.[26] Creating divisions within a targeted society is a common tactic used by invading forces seeking to gain control over local indigenous people. The process often involves techniques that emphasize differences between men and women. Among these techniques are the enlistment of men into newly established militaries and police forces that would answer to colonial authorities and the mandatory schooling of children through which their minds could be colonized. Colonized women, as Frantz Fanon observed in Algeria, were subjected to particular strategies of conquer by the French as a first step toward destroying Algerian society.[27]

Colonial feminist campaigns to save indigenous women from indigenous men throughout the British, French, and Dutch imperialist projects positioned middle-class European women as missionaries of cosmopolitan forms of civility and agents of care. Much of this same logic operates in twenty-first-century technocratic COIN operations. Population-centered counterinsurgency operations in the Global War on Terror sought to reinforce the idea that the U.S.- and NATO-led interventions were humanitarian and had a goal of saving civilian populations in Iraq and Afghanistan. Within COIN operations discourses and militarized forms of aid, references to the civilian population highlighted the saving of women and children. Medical clinics and hospitals became strategic locations for COIN operations aimed at drawing local women into a situation in which they may might be persuaded to offer important information about insurgent activities. As a consequence, far from being neutral safe havens for receiving care, clinics and hospitals became targets for kidnapping, assault, and suicide bombing once insurgents learned that these facilities were being exploited in COIN operations. The ruse of offering care made these women and their children more vulnerable to violence.

As Laleh Khalili explains, compared with the hypermasculinity of battle and combat, counterinsurgency claims to be a "softer" expression of power, concerned more with care than with combat. During the wars in Afghanistan and Iraq, soldier-scholars holding advanced degrees in international relations from major universities promoted counterinsurgency doctrine. Khalili observes the doctrine is "beloved of liberals for its emphasis on 'protection,'" even though its aim is primarily defeating the insurgent "by literally starving him of shelter, food, and medical supplies."[28] COIN doctrine targets the civilian population, and increasingly women, in the remaking of social worlds. Counterinsurgency operations gender space in particular ways, targeting the home, the village, and other areas where women are concentrated. Daily life is studied, subjected to surveillance, and controlled as civilians are "instrumentalized as part and process of the war."[29]

As early as March 2006, Kilcullen endorsed Female Engagement Teams, groups of uniformed U.S. soldiers and marines who were trained to make "culturally aware" contact with Afghan women: "History has taught us that most insurgent fighters are men. But, in traditional societies, women are extremely influential in forming the social networks that insurgents use for support. Co-opting neutral or friendly women, through targeted social and economic programs, builds networks of enlightened self interest that eventually undermines the insurgents. To do this effectively requires your own female counterinsurgents. Win the women, and you *own* the family unit. *Own* the family, and you take a big step forward in mobilizing the population."[30]

During the 2009 troop surge authorized by Obama and carried out under the direction of General Stanley McChrystal before Obama replaced him with Petraeus, counterinsurgency was prioritized as a main strategy that was supposed to convince the Afghan population that the U.S. military was there to protect them. COIN operations funding was initially dedicated mainly to building mosques and roads. In keeping with what COIN planners described as local culture, both of these projects ended up favoring men over women: the mosques were restricted to men, and women were forbidden from using the roads unless escorted by men. When it became obvious that these methods were failing in part because they had overlooked women's needs, a few officers and civilian advisors involved in COIN operations turned their attention to Afghan women, especially those living in locales identified with insurgency.[31] Their hunch was that by providing services to them, women might be able to influence the men in their families and communities to cooperate with the occupying forces. To this end they acquired McChrystal's authorization to train and form Female Engagement Teams (FET).

From the outset, the FET programs assumed that Afghan women would become comfortable talking with armed and uniformed U.S. servicewomen and would welcome their presence, though the founders of the FET program later reported evidence to the contrary.[32] Nevertheless, as the FET program expanded, Marine Corps Major Nina D'Amato, who was also the gender advisor for the Regional Command South West in Afghanistan, framed the COIN operations campaign in terms of changing "the story in a given space." The strategy was a gendered one focused on meeting with local women in villages in order to gather important information about what they most needed as a way to gain their trust. But it was also to implant the narrative that the U.S.-led coalition forces were offering aid, security, and long-term stability. In D'Amato's words, "If you want your narrative entrenched, you focus on the women."[33] And the COIN strategists saw the provision of health care as one of several strategic modes for drawing these women in.

Among the various outreach activities the FET engaged in during the surge of 2009 was serving as intermediaries between doctors from the postinvasion Afghan Ministry of Health (composed mostly of men) and Afghan women and their children. Since the Taliban and insurgent forces were generally unable to provide health care, COIN operations strategists used mobile medical clinics traveling from village to village as a way to appeal to local women by offering to care for them and their children. The FET missions were undermined by a number of factors, notably that U.S. male officers in command did not take the teams seriously, so they lacked sufficient funding to return to locales in order to deepen rapport with Afghan women. Afghan women who came forward with information about men they knew in the Taliban were ignored or jailed by commanders, thus thwarting a fundamental aim of COIN operations. Despite these realities, Cheryl Benard, a political scientist and the lead author of a 2008 RAND paper on women and nation-building, optimistically reported, "Health care operations have been particularly effective in winning local support [in Afghanistan]. On repeated occasions, female patients in health clinics, thankful for care received and motivated to support the new order that provided it, have volunteered valuable tactical information to U.S. forces."[34] Benard, the wife of an Afghan expatriate, Zalmay Khalilzad, Bush's ambassador to the United Nations, omitted a key fact from the 2008 report: since the mobile clinics and other care facilities set up under the auspices of the new Ministry of Health served the dual purpose of drawing women in and of extracting information from them, many became targets for insurgent attacks. Hospitals and clinics were sites of U.S. and NATO military intervention in Iraq and Afghanistan and thus co-opted into spaces of war in the Global War on Terror.[35]

Destroy-and-Build: Replacing Socialized Medicine with Neoliberal Health Care

In Iraq and Afghanistan the health care sector was a primary locus of intervention for refashioning society through a destroy-and-build logic. When the Bush administration set up the Coalition Provisional Authority, one of its main goals was to privatize the previously state-run Iraqi health care system. The CPA reasoned that this transformation would be good for nation-building and for opening Iraq to new multinational business ventures. The process required compelling Iraqi citizens to learn how to be proper neoliberal subjects in a new system that favored reductions in government spending in order to stimulate the private sector and to bring Iraq into the global economy.

A brief historical sketch helps to illustrate how this destroy-and-build process worked in Iraq. The Iran-Iraq War (1980–88), the Persian Gulf War (1990–91), and America's policy of economic sanctions (1990–2003) had compromised the overall health of the Iraqi population. UNICEF analyzed data from two parallel studies and found that between 1991 and 1998, an estimated 400,000 to 500,000 children died due to the Gulf War and economic sanctions.[36] Prior to the 2003 invasion Hussein's Arab socialist Ba'ath Party made the nationalized health care system a priority. This was in part to deal with the adverse health effects caused by events in the previous two decades and also to build party loyalty among medical professionals. When Hussein's regime was toppled in 2003 and the CPA dismantled many existing government institutions, the once-respected national health care system rapidly deteriorated. The CPA banned thousands of Iraqi physicians and nurses from public-sector employment.

Even before the United States invaded Iraq in 2003, the Bush administration explicitly disregarded the anticipated health needs of Iraqi civilians. On January 20, 2003, the administration issued Presidential Directive 24, which moved responsibilities for humanitarian assistance and recovery from the U.S. Department of State and USAID to the U.S. Department of Defense. The State Department and USAID knew that in prolonged warfare, preventable morbidity and mortality could exceed rates of death from violent conflict. Prior to the invasion, USAID signed multimillion-dollar contracts with WHO and UNICEF in anticipation of implementing a postinvasion countrywide program for monitoring health conditions and to provide training in order to serve the most vulnerable populations. However, Bush moved the responsibility of humanitarian aid to the DoD after Secretary of Defense Donald Rumsfeld had assured him that the United States would achieve rapid military success, and therefore a humanitarian crisis would be avoided and there would be no substantial damage to the country's infrastructure. The Bush administration told the U.S. diplomatic corps that they should expect to complete their work in three weeks, shortened from the original three-months departure time they were given earlier.

Directive 24, along with this new timeline, allowed the United States to ignore Articles 55 and 56 of the 4th Geneva Convention, which require rebuilding the public health system of any invaded country. The Department of Defense cut the total budget for humanitarian aid in half, from $4.2 billion, which was recommended by the State Department and USAID, to $2.1 billion. During the invasion Rumsfeld demanded ideological loyalty as a criterion for selection and insisted that the DoD name all postwar appointments for Iraqi ministries. Vice President Dick Cheney consequently removed all of the experienced State Department staff members from their posts in Iraq. Among them was Frederick Burkle Jr., the interim minister of health, a USAID appointee, who was dismissed when he declared Baghdad a public health emergency. With Burkle's dismissal, and as the violent conflict worsened, there was no plan for strategic health recovery or disease monitoring and no active means for measuring mortality and morbidity. Even after Rumsfeld admitted that the conflict required a longer-term military presence and the United States began spending $2.5 billion a week on the war, USAID never received any funds for conducting public health surveillance. Richard Garfield, a public health expert, wrote in 2013, "These lost opportunities, plus the burgeoning insurgency and the scarcity of security services, directly contributed to the chaotic conditions that helped plunge Iraq into an acute-on-chronic public health emergency, which it still remains in today. . . . The only accurate death records are of U.S. and coalition forces. Political decision makers increasingly control public health data, once untouchable. They cannot have it both ways in defining the ground truth: in every war, combatant forces of states and the leaders they serve must be accounted."[37]

During the invasion of Iraq 12 percent of Iraqi hospitals were destroyed. Many medical facilities were looted of equipment and supplies during the first weeks of the war. Vaccination services, control of infectious disease, and tuberculosis treatment were disrupted. As the invasion evolved into a long-term occupation, a sectarian political system, set up under the supervision of the Coalition Provisional Authority, fueled militias and further fomented kidnappings, killings, and the intimidation of public servants, including medical personnel.[38] Clinicians risked their lives on a daily basis just by going to work. The Ministry of Health headquarters in Baghdad was repeatedly attacked.[39] One survey, published in 2012, revealed that between 2003 and 2009, 80 percent of physicians working in Iraqi emergency hospitals had been assaulted by patients or their family members.[40] Between 2003 and 2006 half of the country's 34,000 doctors fled Iraq, 2,000 doctors were killed, and many more became internally displaced, leaving about 9,000 doctors and 15,000 nurses to take care of a population of 28 million.[41] By late 2007 the number of health professionals working in surveyed hospitals in Baghdad had decreased by 78 percent.[42] Those who remained faced insecurity and increasing alienation from their patients, many of whom grew to doubt the neutrality, trustworthiness, and competency of medical staff. The public's distrust of employees of the new Ministry of Health increased as corruption proliferated in the chaotic environment of war and occupation.

Critics of the reconstruction effort pointed out the lack of effective oversight to prevent the misuse or theft of reconstruction funds. In January 2005 Stuart Bowen, the special inspector general for Iraq reconstruction, testified before the U.S. Congress that the Coalition Provisional Authority could not account for how $8 billion of the $37 billion U.S.-administered Development Fund for Iraq was spent. In 2006 the new U.S. special inspector general for Iraq reconstruction, successor to the Coalition Provisional Authority, reported to Congress that many of the funds that were supposed to be spent on reconstruction of infrastructure had been reallocated to "security."[43] Among the many examples of corrupt practices, Abt Associates, a Massachusetts-based consulting firm, was awarded a $43 million contract by the U.S. government in April 2003 to improve the Iraqi Ministry of Health and distribute medical supplies. A USAID audit showed that medical kits intended for six hundred clinics contained damaged or useless equipment and took months to be delivered.[44]

A similar pattern of destruction and corruption occurred in Afghanistan, though the country's pre-invasion medical infrastructure was far less developed than Iraq's. As part of the U.S. plan to rebuild Afghan society, it established a Ministry of Public Health with funding from the World Bank, USAID, and the European Commission. One of the first major programs introduced by the ministry in 2003 was a Basic Package of Health Services (BPHS) to be implemented by government contracts to international and Afghan NGOs. This HMO-like plan provided primary care services in small and rural clinics and was the core of the Afghan health service delivery system at all primary care clinics. It was designed to introduce Afghan citizens to new ways to take responsibility for their health. In 2005 the Essential Package of Hospital Services (EPHS) was established to improve the secondary services for provincial and regional hospitals. The EPHS was concerned with the types of medical services each type of hospital should provide (i.e., staffing, equipment, diagnostic services, medications, and referrals from the BPHS clinics). Despite the fact that these two programs were supposed to provide affordable health care, a survey published in 2012 reported that Afghan households paid for 83 percent of all out-of-pocket health care expenses in 2010.[45]

A similar health management program was established in postinvasion Iraq, again with limited benefits for ordinary people. In addition to the financial burden they faced, wounded or sick Iraqis who sorely needed to visit clinics for treatment of war wounds or other medical emergencies were deterred from doing so because of the physical risk involved. Expectant mothers avoided prenatal care for fear of being injured or killed, which is one factor of several that accounts for why the maternal mortality ratio in Iraq rose from 47 to 84 per 100,000 live births between 2003 and 2006.[46] Patients suffering from chronic conditions and who required regular clinic visits for chemotherapy or dialysis risked their lives to receive treatment.

A column published in 2008 in the *Lancet* harshly criticized the fact that only 4 percent of the $18.4 billion reconstruction budget in Iraq had gone to health care projects by that point and that these projects favored profit-driven private companies aimed at showing short-term achievements rather than long-term health advancements.[47] The author further complained that Iraq's national formulary (its list of medicines) was not written along World Health Organization guidelines but instead was designed to favor European and U.S. suppliers, revealing that concerns for privatized profit were more important to the coalition forces than providing humanitarian aid.

A report issued by Doctors without Borders (DWB) in February 2014 excoriated the U.S.- and NATO-led military intervention in Afghanistan for habitually overemphasizing the achievements of the U.S.-installed Afghan health system while, in practice, neglecting unmet medical needs of Afghans and obstructing their access to clinics and hospitals.[48] The report provided detailed accounts of how military intervention endangered the lives of the people it claimed to be serving. Based on interviews of over eight hundred patients and their caretakers during a six-month period at the four hospitals where DWB teams worked, the researchers found that the ongoing military conflict was "causing widespread disruption to health services, particularly in remote areas." "It is striking how far accounts of ordinary Afghans differ from the prevailing narratives of progress," the writers state. A majority of the people interviewed reported that a combination of insecurity, distance, and high costs made seeking medical care a highly risky undertaking. Many told stories of encountering land mines, checkpoints, roadblocks, and crossfire while on their way to clinics. The expense of traveling long distances to the few existing clinics, coupled with the high price of doctors' fees and medicines, sent many into untenable debt, despite the fact that the new Basic Package of Health Services had promised to provide affordable health care.

"Over the past decade," the report concluded, "decisions on where and how to provide assistance have too often been based on desires for stabilization, force protection or 'winning hearts and minds,' at the expense of adequately addressing people's most pressing needs." It complained that, as casualties mounted due to an upswing in violent attacks, clinics and hospitals were being "misappropriated" for nonmedical purposes, such as voter registration and COIN operations, thus "damaging the perception of health centers as neutral spaces to provide medical care, and putting the lives of health workers and patients in danger."[49] The report concluded that, through the U.S. military's COIN operations' doctrinal framework, aid provision became threat-based rather than needs-based, operating as part of the "quick impact projects" that were intended to appeal to the population in certain insurgency-affected areas even though other locales were also in need of basic health care. When over half of the population had little or no access to basic health care,[50] the claims of progress were, in the view of the DWB report's authors, fanciful and mainly aimed at satisfying what large donor organizations such as the World Bank, USAID, and the European Commission wanted to hear.

A not-so-hidden agenda of the Bush administration's nation-building plans for Afghanistan and Iraq was refashioning the populations of those lands into people who would take responsibility for their health and become what Katherine E. Kenny has referred to as the neoliberal *Homo oeconomicus*.[51] The World Bank in the early 1990s posited this new type of subject in the context of austerity programs imposed on regions in the Global South to pay back debts to the World Bank and the IMF. What kind of subject was needed to repay the mounting debt resulting from development programs devised by the IMF and the World Bank? A nominally healthy and well-disciplined subject who could be educated for private-sector employment and whose efforts would generate revenues for paying off the nation's debt. This neoliberal political rationality conceives of the human as primarily an economic agent whose life is valued according to metrics that measure health in terms of human capital and thus define health as a site of investment. The neoconservative ideologues that urged the United States to go to war with Iraq in 2003 imagined that the postinvasion societies of Iraq as well as Afghanistan would be places to cultivate *Homo oeconomicus*. Subjects would invest in their own health and self-improvement in order to contribute to the economy in the rebuilding of a destroyed country. Such a subject should be grateful for being given the gift of freedom and should be future-oriented in self-optimizing ways with minimal provisions from the state, an entrepreneur of the self. The destroy-and-build strategy that unleashed catastrophic violence in Iraq and Afghanistan was enabled by a cavalier attitude expressed by Bush, Cheney, and Rumsfeld that the populations of both those nations would greet invaders with open arms and readily comply with building the new nation. Disguised as care, the campaign to remake societies and subjects through violent destruction was informed by a hubristic economization of life.

Exploiting the Pretense of Care in Covert Operations

As the wars dragged on, what little belief people in those regions had that health care facilities were neutral diminished after the revelation that medical care had been co-opted in the covert military operation that led to the assassination of Osama bin Laden in Abbottabad, Pakistan, in May 2011. Following his death, global news media reported that the U.S. government had used a vaccination campaign for gathering intelligence that might lead to his whereabouts. Officially referred to as a hepatitis C vaccination program, the CIA operation in Abbottabad was intended to secretly gather DNA from bin Laden's relatives in order to confirm that he was in the area. When the program was exposed, it further eroded local trust in aid workers, deepening the suspicion of many Pakistanis toward medical clinics throughout the country and providing a tool that the Taliban leadership exploited, declaring a series of fatwas against vaccination programs. The Pakistani government was furious at the CIA's violation of Pakistani sovereignty. In May 2012 Dr. Shakil Afridi, who was in charge of the CIA's Abbottabad program, was convicted of high treason and sentenced to thirty-three years in prison. Though originally it seemed that the charge of treason was based on his participation in the bin Laden raid, the Pakistani court clarified that it was because of his alleged ties to a local warlord from the banned Islamist group Lashkar-e-Islam. Afridi was held in solitary confinement and abandoned by the United States in deference to Pakistan, a key player in facilitating U.S. peace talks with the Afghan Taliban.[52]

By the time of Afridi's conviction, militants had killed at least sixteen Pakistani health workers. In June 2012 the Taliban leadership and several Islamic clerics issued a fatwa banning polio workers from vaccinating people in Waziristan as long as the United States continued to conduct drone attacks in the region.[53] Polio eradication experts feared that the collapse of vaccination programs that employed 225,000 vaccinators in Pakistan, where the disease was not fully contained, would lead to an outbreak of cases.[54]

The killing of local health workers and volunteers by Islamist groups prompted deans from thirteen prominent public health schools in the United States to write a letter to the White House on January 8, 2012, demanding that the U.S. government stop using "sham vaccination" programs for the purposes of gaining military intelligence.[55] Over a year after the letter was sent to President Obama, CIA spokesman Dean Boyd defended the Abbottabad vaccination campaign in a statement made to ABC News, insisting that the program was not "fake" because, while it was used for gathering biometric data for intelligence purposes, it was also a health care provider, vaccinating local children. The program could have succeeded, he insisted, if the Pakistani government hadn't arrested and convicted Afridi, actions that prevented the children from being fully immunized. Boyd went on to state that the CIA had been directed in August 2013 to "make no operational use of [the] vaccination program, which includes vaccination workers." He remarked that "long-standing extremist claims that foreign vaccination programs are spy operations run by Western governments" stood in the way of successful vaccination programs abroad, similar to other obstacles, like "myths that vaccinations cause sterility or HIV."[56]

But as the public health school deans predicted, the CIA's exploitation of vaccination campaigns led to a backlash against immunization in Pakistan and hence to an increase in cases of polio. The U.S. Centers for Disease Control and Prevention estimated that over 350,000 children were prevented from being immunized starting in 2011. As a consequence, between 2013 and 2014 the cases of polio increased by 60 percent in Pakistan, for a total of 150 patients, with several cases imported to neighboring Afghanistan and war-torn Syria.[57]

Because of the physical destruction of clinics and hospitals, the deaths or refugee departures of vast numbers of medical professionals, and the sheer danger and financial expense of traveling through battle zones to the few remaining clinics, women, children, and men suffering from war injuries in these locales died in greater numbers and at faster rates than U.S. soldiers afflicted by the same or lesser assaults.[58]

Bio-inequality is evident in war itself: some lives are to be taken (the enemy), and some to be protected (one's own). However, wars that are conducted in the name of "rescue," as well as preemptive wars, are rationalized in the name of humanity at large within a distinctly cosmopolitan understanding of the global political space. The rights-bearing cosmopolitan liberal subject in this discourse is posited as superior to those belonging to groups who are assumed to be incapable of self-governing and therefore who are deemed to be subject either to rescue or discipline, to being killed, or to being abandoned to die. The calculus posited by wars fought in the name of humanity measures who is and who is not worthy of life. Such wars cast the enemy as a racial Other.

The benefits of biomedicine are selectively distributed. In the case of wounded bodies, military medical personnel are charged with caring for their own. Any care they provide for civilian men, women, or children they encounter in the war zone is secondary to the care they are expected to provide for U.S. military personnel. Calculations of the value of life are made along a fault line dividing friend from foe, despite the rhetoric of rescue and the gift of freedom. In addition, in very practical terms, calculations of the value of life are made by military medical personnel, often under conditions of duress, in which a physician must decide who should be cared for first. Should it be the one whose injury is most life-threatening or the one who might be able to return to duty if sufficiently treated? These calculations are situated in a larger framework within which military operations are structured ostensibly around what Eyal Weizman refers to as the *lesser evil principle* that pertains to military rules of engagement and to international human rights law. This principle of proportionality calls for calculating how to achieve one's military objectives without "unnecessary use of force" against an enemy and with minimal risk to one's own forces. It is the doctrine according to which the Obama administration justified use of armed unmanned aerial vehicles in targeted assassinations. Surgical strikes that minimize collateral damage and remove threats are based on calculations and predictions concerning the value of life. Predictions are never certain, so calculations of risk always involve weighing options and hedging risks. Calculations of acceptable violence are about speculation.[59]

U.S.-led military interventions in Afghanistan and Iraq were promoted by the Bush administration and its supporters under the dual banner of self-defense and humanitarianism, staking the wars' legitimacy on moral grounds especially when international law provided no legal grounds for them. Yet the military logic of minimizing risk to one's own forces and maximizing risks to one's enemy operated. The *Lancet* reported that during the first fifteen months after the invasion of Iraq, the U.S.-led coalition forces lost about 1,040 troops, while the Iraqis lost 100,000 civilians, most of them women and children.[60] If the U.S.-led coalition forces did not intend to kill civilians, but these deaths were the result of unfortunate collateral damage resulting from the coalition's strategy to keep their own losses to a minimum, then it would appear that the life of one U.S. soldier was worth one thousand times the life of a civilian Iraqi, whom the United States and its coalition were fighting to protect and defend.

The United States compensated a small fraction of the Afghan and Iraqi families who lost loved ones, and only in cases where fault was found.[61] As Emily Gilbert and Corey Ponder argue, war-related compensation was part of a security apparatus "that is mobilized not simply as an act of generosity or humanitarianism, but to restore the efficient circulation of economies and the population."[62] The lesser compensation offered to Afghan and Iraqi families compared to that offered to families of injured or killed American service members reflects Foucault's account of biopolitics, in which power works "to foster life or to disallow it to the point of death."[63] Americans received reparative compensation to restore the economic life of their families, while Afghans and Iraqis were placed in a condition of slow death, abandoned to die, subjected to the constitutive violence of biopower that works alongside the optimization of life, which, Tania Li writes, "consigns large numbers of people to live short and limited lives."[64]

SYNOPSIS

The nexus that entangles biomedicine with war is rooted in fantasies of security and care that animate institutions and practices of everyday life in our total war society and that are enacted in America's military operations of invasion, occupation, and targeted assassinations. I have argued that domestic and national security, counterinsurgency operations, and allegories of medical intervention are part of a larger disciplinary corpus to remake societies and manage populations according to a technocratic investment in "advancement," through which new kinds of proper citizens are supposed to be produced. Attachments to cherished and mystifying narratives of technoscientific progress and biomedical advancement have authorized violence in the name of necessary sacrifices that sort the worthy from the unworthy through racializing tactics that target some bodies for protection, some for reform, and some for elimination. Sentiments of fear and enmity propel an ever-expanding security apparatus in a complex relationship to the cruel optimism of popular faith in biomedical salvation.

TWO

Promises of Polytrauma

On Regenerative Medicine

In 2010, *60 Minutes*, then in its fourth decade of broadcasts, introduced its audience to Dr. Anthony Atala in a feature story covering the emergent field of regenerative medicine. A highly regarded clinical researcher in the area of tissue engineering and cellular therapeutics, the Peruvian native showed the crew around the Wake Forest Institute for Regenerative Medicine, where his team was experimenting with cultivating cells, tissues, and organs to restore severely injured veterans' bodies. The Institute, based at Wake Forest University School of Medicine and the Wake Forest Baptist Medical Center, consisted of two research consortiums when it was established in 2008. In 2013 it became part of the larger Armed Forces Institute of Regenerative Medicine (AFIRM) II's Warrior Restoration Consortium, which consisted of researchers at thirty-one hospitals around the United States (many based at Research I universities) conducting clinical studies to develop therapies for treating wounds. According to a press release of the Institute, the academic-industry team of AFIRM "will work with health professionals at the U.S. Army Institute of Surgical Research and Walter Reed National Military Medical Center to develop new treatments for wounded soldiers."[1]

Atala and other researchers in regenerative medicine work at the intersections of war medicine and bioengineering, where the damages of war spur innovation. Military veterans who are the patients and research

The cost of this war in Afghanistan, for civilians and military, has been exceptionally high. But I do believe some good will come out of so much suffering, and that because of what we've learnt, future lives will be saved.

—**MICHAEL MOSLEY**, BBC science journalist, "Miracles of War: How Front-Line Injuries Inform Modern Medicine" subjects of regenerative medicine suffer from polytrauma, a recently coined term of art used in civilian emergency and war medicine to classify patients with complex and often grave injuries affecting different organ systems. Biomedical salvation infused the story of regenerative medicine research and patients featured in the 60 Minutes segment. Their wound narratives and injured bodies were central to news about the promises of bioengineered organs, tissues, and limbs. Research on regenerative medicine, seeded with taxpayers' dollars in public-private partnerships, expanded substantially with the return of hundreds of wounded troops diagnosed with polytrauma.

This chapter centers on regenerative medicine and explores the meaning of *war-generated polytrauma*. Media coverage of this catastrophic condition offers a revealing example of what I am calling narratives of biomedical salvation that attach ordinary Americans to war. As thousands of severely injured troops returned from combat in Afghanistan and Iraq, journalists portrayed regenerative medicine as key for salvaging beneficial knowledge from war's ruins. War, they acknowledged, was awful, but it could give rise to miracles. A cruel optimism is prompted by this logic: terribly traumatized patients faced a double bind in which the scientific dream of regeneration required their cooperation in exhausting rehabilitation regimens that were only partially successful. The moral authority of these stories centered on the possibility of miraculous regeneration and the saving of lives. The coverage melded grateful patriotism with faith in technoscientific innovation. Feeling remorse for the suffering who risked their lives for the nation's defense, viewers were encouraged to understand war as having the potential to strengthen emotional bonds, generate hope, build dreams, and reconstitute bodies. Gestures of care and compassion were dramatized in these narratives, forging attachments among those who have not been in combat, those who have, and those with expertise to take care of war-generated polytrauma survivors.

Biomedical logics that emphasize an ethic of care in the wake of combat injuries serve as ideological mystifications that rationalize war—that make war thinkable through what can be redeemed from it. But for it to be redeemed, war requires the affective investment of citizens in the hope that it will open new horizons for knowledge such that future lives may be saved. Biomedical logics are anticipatory, enlisting the future as a salve for the suffering of the present.[2] The condition of war and the biomedical response to it prepare us for the saving of abstract future lives, warranting affective and financial investments in the speculative realm of biotechnology. Patients whose injuries are deemed significant are pressed into duty (again) to help realize the dream of regeneration.

Polytrauma is referred to as a "signature injury" in military medical discourses. I argue that it indexes a particular kind of *woundscape* and requires particular reading practices to interpret the significance that is attributed to the injury both in biomedical and geopolitical terms. I borrow the idiom *woundscape* from the audio artist Gregory Whitehead, who coined the term as a way of talking about serious injuries that create "a complex and multilayered woundscape."[3] The idea originated from Whitehead's reflections on being one of eight people involved in a near fatal car accident when he was sixteen. In *Display Wounds*, he takes up the role of a "vulnerologist" faced with the impossibility of translating the literal meaning of individual wounds, especially in contexts of catastrophic collisions or mass killings. "The practice of the vulnerologist," Whitehead writes, "is oriented more towards getting the *feel* of the wound, sensing its quality, sensing the deeper implications of its experience." For my purposes, war-generated polytrauma is more than a name for an injury; it is also a concept-effect of the mutual provocation between war-generated violence and healing practices. As a woundscape, war-generated polytrauma gives rise to fantasies of miraculous healing and dreams of acquiring better knowledge about biological systems through reading wounds. These fantasies and dreams are premised on the condition of surviving horrible violence. The task of the vulnerologist of war-generated polytrauma is to convey a sense of what elements bring this complex wound into being. This would include the weaponry, the historical and cultural context of its emergence, and the elaboration of its qualities in biomedical discourse and scientific knowledge production. The woundscape of polytrauma encompasses these dynamics as well as the stories generated about the injury that appear in popular media. I attempt in this chapter to write as a vulnerologist.

The diagnosis of war-generated polytrauma is a historically specific codification that reflects the convergence of particular weapons systems, battle tactics, medical subdisciplines, and complex treatment methods. I analyze the meaning of war-generated polytrauma by examining clinics and laboratories, experts, products, and patients introduced to the public in media stories focused on novel ways in which medical knowledge is advanced as a consequence of war. I discuss the biomedical logics of salvation that frame news about cutting-edge research in bioengineering. I describe scenarios in which the promise of regeneration is offered to individual patients whose injuries are regarded as significant and also to the larger audience bearing witness to the technoscientific wonders of regenerating life. The wounds of *significantly injured* patients—American troops—prompt an indebtedness whereby the nation owes twice for the sacrifices made: once for the wound acquired while serving the nation and again for the new knowledge that can be derived from medical treatment of the warrior's suffering. Ordinary people become attached to war through the hope they invest in biomedical promises that are prompted by the severe injuries sustained by returning veterans. And biomedicine deepens its attachment to war by counting on its damage to develop new knowledge. This kind of attachment does not question the morality of war itself.

THE SIGNATURE INJURY OF POLYTRAUMA

Journalists reporting on regenerative therapies for wounded veterans repeat a script frequently told by physicians and by historians of military medicine: that each modern war has its signature injury that results from specific weapons systems and combat strategies.[4] According to the conventional narrative, medical research on signature injuries gives rise to innovations that will be valuable for saving future lives. *Signature* injuries—as their central metaphor suggests—leave recognizable marks to be read. They can be analyzed using semiotic-forensic tools to specify their place in the interwoven histories of weapons technology, warfare, and life science. Such an analysis brings to light a matrix of dynamic elements: weapons, targets, physical locations, bodies, sentiments, military strategies, medical procedures, diagnostic terminologies, rehabilitative therapies, and geopolitical histories. In this respect wounding is a situated act of signification that produces the signature injury, which can, in turn, be interpreted to clarify such details as ballistic force and the damage it does. The injury can be read for evidence of the entanglements of medical knowledge with military strategy. It indexes larger geopolitical dynamics that make certain types of wounds possible. The central metaphor of the signature evokes the matter of significance. In this sense the term *signature injury* is also evaluative. What counts as a significant injury, and whose injuries are significant? As we will see, some peoples' injuries are valued and innovations to treat them are heralded, while the injuries of others are not.

Polytrauma has been designated as one of the signature injuries of the Global War on Terror. It is defined as damage to more than one organ or physiological system. While polytrauma can result from accidents and injuries not caused by war, it is classified in war-related medicine as an umbrella condition that encompasses a collection of recently codified and proliferating "blast wound" designations. Traumatic brain injury, compartment syndrome, crush syndrome, and dismounted complex blast injury are some of these new designations, each hailing particular kinds of specialists and each clustering together specific symptoms that are caused by detonating devices. Clinicians diagnose war-generated polytrauma in patients who, as a result of exposure to explosions, suffer from several or all of the following: head injuries, loss of vision and hearing, nerve damage, vertigo, multiple bone fractures, shattered teeth, lost limbs, broken ear drums, metabolic derangement, internal bleeding, asphyxiation, infections, burn wounds, persistent unhealed wounds, and, often, a range of emotional or behavioral problems. These are the blasts' horrible signatures.

Because of the complexity of their injuries, patients diagnosed with polytrauma require a variety of expensive treatments, which, ideally, are coordinated by interdisciplinary teams of clinicians and therapists. Each patient needs a personalized plan of care, administered over a long period of recovery, often lifelong. Some require the help of rehabilitation therapists, speech therapists, neurologists, dentists, audiologists, ophthalmologists, urologists, psychiatrists, orthopedic surgeons, or ear, nose, and throat doctors. Increasingly too, scientists and engineers with expertise in materials science, regenerative tissue cultivation, artificial intelligence, and robotics design participate in war-generated polytrauma research.

War-generated polytrauma among American troops is a consequence of the proliferation of improvised explosive devices, land mines, and rocket-propelled grenades exploited by insurgent groups. But the syndrome came into being also because of certain advancements related to survivability from severe injuries. Over the past four major wars in which the United States has participated, rates of survivability have increased. Thirty percent of American service members injured in combat during World War II died. During the war in Vietnam, 24 percent of those injured died. The fatality rate dropped to around 10 percent during the early years of the wars in Afghanistan and Iraq. Although the percentage of wounded troops has not really changed since the U.S. Revolutionary War, the difference now is that troops wear greater protective gear and the infrastructure supporting emergency combat medicine facilitates rapid evacuation and treatment by highly trained triage medics.[5] Forward operating clinics and emergency medical teams now have blood-clotting products that keep severely wounded patients alive who in previous wars would have "bled out." But having survived death, polytrauma patients present novel challenges and face grueling rehabilitation regimens. They populate a woundscape in which crude devices deployed by minimally trained ragtag militias cause extreme damage while advanced technology keeps the injured alive. Their suffering is profound.

During the wars in Afghanistan and Iraq, patients were transported to the handful of special polytrauma centers recently established in the United States. The severity of a patient's brain injury determined the course of care. If a veteran no longer had the ability to think, learn, or remember, the regimen of care focused on feeding, toileting, and comforting the patient. If a veteran still had cognitive ability, he or she was guided toward more complex rehabilitative activities, such as learning to speak or to walk with prosthetic legs. For many, exposure to explosions caused severe psychological distress and impaired their ability to concentrate, retain information, or process experiences.

The term *blast wounds* conjures up images of visibly apparent, severely injured bodies. But exposure to blasts also causes injuries that are not immediately evident. The U.S. Veterans Administration reported that between 2002 and 2011 more than 60 percent of service members deployed to Iraq and Afghanistan reported some degree of blast exposure, many suffering from mild traumatic brain injury (TBI), also known as concussion or "closed-head injury." A Congressional Budget Office report from 2012 noted that mild TBI accounted for 90 percent of all TBI cases among active-duty service members.[6] Common symptoms included difficulty thinking clearly or concentrating, irritability, sadness, nervousness, anxiety, disordered sleep, headaches, blurred vision, dizziness, sensitivity to light or noise, slurred speech, numbness, nausea, balance problems, and feeling tired.[7] Patients often experienced difficulty thinking clearly or concentrating. Among those with no visible wounds the diagnosis arose from observing the patient's behavior or listening to the patient's account of symptoms. A fundamental problem with the diagnosis of mild TBI is that many of its symptoms are shared with other conditions, chiefly posttraumatic stress. This made postdeployment screening of returning veterans for mild TBI, which the Department of Veterans Affairs began to require in 2007, more of an approximation than a definitive method.[8]

Blast-related TBIs are generally more severe than head injuries caused by vehicular collisions or athletic accidents. The explosive detonation intensifies the severity of brain damage. Research reported in 2006 from the Defense and Veterans Brain Injury Center at Walter Reed Army Medical Center indicated that patients suffering from blast-related closed-head injuries were more likely to have seizures than patients with closed-head injuries that were not caused by blasts. Those diagnosed with mild TBI were more likely to have an acute stress reaction or posttraumatic stress disorder (PTSD) than people who sustained mild concussions under non-war-related circumstances. Mild TBI patients who remained conscious during the blast suffered symptoms of chronic hypervigilance, such as startling easily and experiencing a persistent sense of insecurity.[9] The circumstances of war exacerbate the suffering.

EXPERT DISCOURSE ON POLYTRAUMA

The diagnosis of polytrauma is constructed within a woundscape in which scientific discourse delineates types of detonating devices and describes the temporal trajectory of their damaging effects. The tone of the discourse is methodical, objectifying, and impersonal. Its structure is symptomatically bullet-point-like.

According to this discourse, when a conventional bomb is detonated, it sends a blast wave that emanates from one point and consists of two main stages. First, a high-pressure shock wave projects energy out from the point of origin, causing overpressurization of the air. The primary stage involves an implosion caused when gas pockets contract as the blast waves travel through tissue and then re-expand, causing multiple miniature internal explosions. Also at this stage the body experiences abrupt acceleration followed by equally abrupt deceleration, as the body and internal organs are thrown in one direction by the initial blast and then in another by meeting a solid object such as a wall or pavement. The high pressure of the primary stage causes shock waves that damage ears, eyes, lungs, the gastrointestinal tract, the central nervous system, and the cardiovascular system. The most common injury is the rupturing of the tympanic membrane, manifesting in deafness, tinnitus, and vertigo. The high pressure may also rupture the globe of the eyeball and result in retinitis (inflammation of the retina) or hyphema (a buildup of blood between the cornea and the iris). The central nervous system is vulnerable under such high pressure to barotraumas caused by abrupt changes in air pressure and gas embolism (air bubbles that block a vein or artery). Bone fractures are common. The intensity of overpressurization causes internal injuries to spleens, livers, and kidneys.[10]

> *Vulnerology: Boom! Damaged organs and devastated physiologies.*
> *Can't hear. Dizzy. Shattered bones. Bleeding inside.*
> *Ballistic metrics. Cold hard facts.*
> *The dispassionate discourse continues.*

The injury's primary stage is followed by a blast wind that reverses the air motion back toward the blast, causing a vacuum effect. This results in underpressurization, which damages organs, especially organs with air-fluid interfaces such as lungs. The blast wind propels fragments and bodies, which leads to blunt and penetrating injuries. As objects—including bodies—are propelled through space, debris and shrapnel puncture the skin, causing tissue and organ damage. Infected or partially severed limbs must be amputated. This secondary stage can also result in open-brain and eye injuries.

> *Vulnerology: debris, shrapnel, organ damage, amputation, infection,*
> *can't breathe, can't see, suffocating, bleeding*
> *a vacuum effect*
> *The explanation continues.*

Weapons categorized as enhanced-blast explosive devices are more damaging than conventional bombs because they set off a primary explosion that is followed by a secondary blast. Lockheed Martin holds the patent for this type of device.[11] They are designed to penetrate tunnels, caves, and walls, using blast waves that can travel around corners and with thermobaric properties (thermal radiation and use of oxygen) to create a rapid, localized energy release. They are highly destructive when detonated in confined environments because they consume all the available oxygen and generate a sustained blast wave. They use thinner munitions casings than conventional blast warheads. Most of the released energy results in a fireball and a blast or shock wave. The result is that a high-pressure wave radiates through a much wider area than with conventional bombs by extending the overpressurization stage and intensifying the total energy that is transmitted by the blast. When either conventional or enhanced bombs are detonated inside buildings or vehicles, the high-pressure waves are intensified and cause eccentric patterns of injury.

Vulnerology: Fireball. Shock wave. Trapped in a tunnel. No oxygen.
High-pressure
Eardrums shattered
Lockheed Martin

Explosions also cause tertiary blast injuries, when the person is thrown against the ground or crushed by a collapsing structure. Children, because they weigh less than adults, are particularly susceptible to these injuries. In this family of injuries is crush syndrome, characterized by metabolic derangement unleashed by being crushed. Damaged tissue causes the victim to release myoglobin, urates, potassium, and phosphates. Renal failure can result from the retention of potassium beyond that released by the damaged muscle. A related diagnosis is compartment syndrome, caused by compression that a damaged, edematous (accumulation of excess fluid) muscle exerts within its elastic sheath, leading to restriction in blood supply, swelling, and local tissue death if untreated, and usually occurring in the extremities. It can be detected from a level of pain that is out of proportion to the injury.

Vulnerology: Metabolic derangement. Crushed.
Collapsing walls. Compression.
Swelling. Kidney failure.
Extreme pain. Child flying.

Explosion-related injuries entail radiation poisoning, asphyxiation, and thermal burns from the bomb itself or from the resulting fire. Napalm or radioactive materials used in incendiary bombs are a common cause of these injuries.

Vulnerology: Choking. Burning. From the inside out.
Can't breathe
Skin is melting

Dismounted complex blast injury (DCBI), a subset of polytrauma, is the U.S. military's technical classification assigned to injuries sustained by troops on foot patrol who step on a land mine or encounter an IED.

The U.S. Army established a DCBI Task Force in 2010, when incidents of this sort increased. The diagnosis typically involves patients who have lost at least one leg and experienced severe injury to another extremity while also sustaining wounds to the pelvis, abdomen, and/or urogenital organs. DCBI patients are prone to infection, so they often require longer and higher doses of medication. Sexual dysfunction and fertility problems are common among patients with genital damage, requiring experts in these fields to participate in rehabilitation. Patients suffer a predominance of "high-thigh amputations" and genital injuries specifically associated with dismounted patrolling. Because IEDs are often buried in the ground, when they explode, the blast is directed upward and causes damage to the feet, legs, and external genitalia first.

> Vulnerology: High-thigh amputations. Genital injuries. Pelvic pain.
> Can't pee properly. Sexual dysfunction. Loss of identity.
> The rates of DCBI increased substantially during the massive U.S.
> troop surges ordered by Bush and Obama.[12]

The dramatic increase in genitourinary injuries led one war journalist covering the wars in Iraq and Afghanistan to declare it a signature injury.[13] The DCBI designation was intended by military physicians to provide insight into the specific causes and appropriate treatments for blast wounds due to certain tactical maneuvers and war-fighting goals, especially those associated with counterinsurgency campaigns that involve circulating on foot among the local population.[14]

Over these past few pages I have attempted to convey *a sense* of the injury of war-generated polytrauma. The dispassionate quality of the diagnostic terminology that explains the injury attaches war to medicine while detaching the injury from specific bodies and lives that it afflicts. This is typical of clinical discourse and not unique to military medicine. But compared with the heart-rending portrayals of veterans going through rehabilitation that appeal to audiences of shows like *60 Minutes*, the expert discourse on blast wounds feels particularly alienating. The U.S. military deployed many of these explosive devices in populated locales. Women, children, and noncombatant men suffered from blast wounds in numbers that far exceeded the injuries of American troops. Yet their stories were not featured in the accounts of regenerative medicine's promise for treating polytrauma. This omission is an absent presence in the woundscape of blast injuries.

Receiving a diagnosis of polytrauma is of course contingent upon the patient's survival. This fact, together with media publicity about polytrauma teams and regenerative medicine, solidified an image of the typical polytrauma patient as an American veteran. Absent from this publicity were Afghan or Iraqi civilians who suffered wounds medically identical to or more devastating than those of American troops. Children injured by blasts tended to have higher injury severity scores and greater mortality rates than adult patients with polytrauma.[15] Aerial bombardments by the U.S.-led coalition dropping white phosphorous bombs, daisy cutter bombs, and cluster bombs killed people before they could receive emergency care. That the image of the typical polytrauma patient was an American soldier or marine and not an Iraqi or Afghan was not due solely to an inherent racism in media coverage about biomedical advances. It was because an overwhelming number of civilians succumbed to blast wounds. The hope staked in polytrauma medicine depends on severely wounded bodies that survive. In order to advance, regenerative medicine needed badly wounded bodies, bodies that would have bled out in earlier wars.

By 2014 the overwhelming number of polytrauma patients being treated in U.S. military or Veterans Administration hospitals were men, most of them in the noncommissioned and enlisted ranks of the Marine Corps and U.S. Army.[16] Many served in infantry, convoy, or explosives ordnance disposal units in Iraq or Afghanistan. Patriotic heteronormativity framed the typical patient's portrait in media stories about polytrauma. The central character was usually a young man who, we were told, volunteered for military service following 9/11. He was usually depicted in a series of before, during, and after photographs that emphasized his vitality and strength prior to the injury, his disfigurement and frailty following it, and his unsteady but determined course of therapeutic rehabilitation. His injured body marked the sacrifice that was to be honored. His rehabilitation was painstaking and demanded hope. Viewers were introduced to care providers and to family and friends—concerned girlfriends or wives and parents, siblings, and buddies—whose patience, devotion, and love were central to the process of rehabilitation. The cost of his rehabilitation was never mentioned, nor was much said about the working conditions of those who were involved in caring for him.[17] The woundscape of war-generated polytrauma was shaped by hegemonic representations that emphasized patients' individual will, resilience, and determination to become well again. The American public was hailed to strengthen an attachment to biomedical solutions to make up for the sacrifices wounded men made for the nation. This would take a considerable amount of money. Rather than questioning the morality of the wars, media stories and congressional debates about allocating funds for regenerative medicine focused on what these suffering veterans deserved. While investigative journalists unearthed scandalous neglect and mistreatment of veterans in VA and military hospitals, feel-good stories about the promising horizon of regenerative medicine offered a counterpoint in the register of biomedical salvation.

POLYTRAUMA AND BIOMEDICAL SALVATION

As cases of war-related polytrauma increased, Congress allocated funding to establish facilities where multidisciplinary care could be coordinated with biomedical research trials. As early as 2004 the U.S. Central Command set up a Joint Theater Trauma System aimed at improving trauma care on the battlefield. In the following year Congress mandated that the Veterans Administration establish specialized clinics for treating and, when possible, rehabilitating polytrauma patients. By 2007 four major VA polytrauma centers were operating around the United States, where the average length of stay was thirty-two days, after which the majority of patients were typically discharged to their family's home, assuming they had such support in their lives. Each center had between twelve and eighteen inpatient beds and provided acute interdisciplinary evaluation, medical management, and rehabilitation.[18] Each had a transitional rehabilitation program that assisted patients suffering from PTSD and substance abuse and that provided vocational counseling. The centers' Emerging Consciousness Program treated patients in comatose states with experimental drugs to stimulate brain activity. In addition to the VA facilities, military prosthetic and rehabilitation centers were established at Fort Sam Houston, Texas, the Military Advanced Training Center in Washington, D.C., and Balboa Naval Medical Center in San Diego. In 2006 the Department of Defense implemented an evidence-based Blast Injury Research Program and the Joint Trauma Analysis and Prevention of Injury in Combat Program to identify "threat vulnerabilities" by coordinating relevant work across the branches of service. The Army Center for Enhanced Performance (ACEP), originally established at the U.S. Military Academy at West Point, was incorporated into the larger care apparatus for polytrauma patients, whose mission was to provide "a systematic educational and development process to enhance adaptive thinking, mental agility, and self-regulation skills essential to the pursuit of overall personal strength, professional excellence, and the Warrior Ethos," also known as "resilience enhancement."[19] By the tenth anniversary of the events of 9/11, war-related polytrauma had given rise to an extensive network of new initiatives within the U.S. military dedicated to contending with the complicated effects of surviving profound injury. The "Warrior Ethos" terminology of resilience and self-improvement echoed with the growing hegemony of post-Reagan ideas that fetishized the self-made entrepreneur who confronted challenges with an ambitious spirit of competition to come out on top. There is nothing you cannot do if you put your mind to it: cruel optimism in perhaps its most concentrated form. This logic lionized patients who fought hard to recover. It had little patience for those who gave up. As suicide rates among returning veterans soared, the selective media focus of 60 Minutes on a few severely injured men hard at work to make themselves well again obfuscated the anguish of so many men and women returning home from war.

As the number of polytrauma patients increased, starting in 2008 the Department of Defense began allocating money for biomedical research to contend with the special needs of this group. Government contracts were awarded to private for-profit clinics, materials manufacturers, academic institutions, and nongovernmental nonprofit entities. In 2012 the army reported improvement in triage procedures, evacuation logistics, pain management, and burn support. It lauded DoD-funded research for yielding new blood-clotting products, portable sonography, and neurally integrated prosthetic limbs.[20] The experimental field of regenerative medicine was especially promising in the view of the Department of Defense.

Regenerative medicine researchers engineer tissue in vitro in order to regenerate organs and replace damaged or missing skin. The field became a focal point of the military's translational research that applied promising laboratory experiments to clinical treatment. Media stories about innovations in regenerative medicine link military medicine to new sectors of the biotechnology industry. I have chosen a specific story in order to illustrate how the idea of regeneration—in which engineered cells stimulate the body to regrow tissue—resonates with biomedical salvation.[21] So back to Dr. Anthony Atala's laboratory we go.

SCENARIO: SALVATION THROUGH REGENERATION

In the 60 *Minutes* segment from 2010, Atala leads a seasoned journalist around the Institute for Regenerative Medicine, pointing out one of his team's accomplishments: a bladder made from cultivated tissue.[22] Other works in progress are a bioengineered heart valve, a biomanufactured ear, and a mouse liver, all made from regenerated cells in a process that, we are told, can take only six to eight weeks. "The possibilities really are endless," Atala tells CBS's Morley Safer, whose voice-over narration cites Atala's as the largest laboratory in the world dedicated to the bioengineering of body parts.

Regenerative medicine, 60 *Minutes* tells us, is a new horizon of experimental research that aims to provide a solution to the problem of the shortage of organs available for transplants. Atala's procedure involves isolating a particular organ's cells and then multiplying enough of them to coat a three-dimensional mold of the missing or injured body part, one layer at a time, "like baking a layer cake," he tells Safer. "But," Safer asks, "how do those cells know—it's a really stupid question, I understand—but how do the bladder cells know they should be functioning as bladder cells?" "The cells know exactly what to do," Atala responds confidently. "Every single cell in your body has all the genetic information to create a whole new you. So if you place that cell in the right environment, it'll be programmed to do what it's supposed to do." The segment sidesteps the controversial subject of human embryonic stem cells, whose high value for regenerative medicine resides in their pluripotency—the capability to be cultivated into any tissue or organ of the body.

Atala is no stranger to the political battles over human embryonic stem cell research. He worked around the federal ban on funding embryonic stem cell research for years, relying on support from Geron, a private biotech company, dating back to 1998. In exchange the company held exclusive rights to Atala's findings. Geron, founded in 1990 and based in Menlo Park, California, was financed by venture capital and, as Melinda Cooper notes, by 2003 "offered little more than the hope of future revenues from its patent portfolio." Geron began trading publicly on the NASDAQ in 1996, but its products never generated a profit. With a name that signals its focus on cellular aging and cellular immortalization, Geron offered products for targeting the enzyme that stimulates cancerous cells to replicate immortally, for deriving and scaling up undifferentiated embryonic stem cell lines, and for differentiating these lines into therapeutically useful cells.

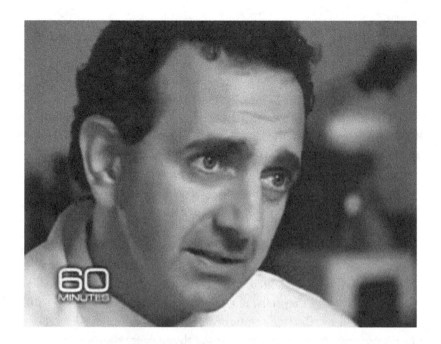

To make up for an absence of profits from these products, Geron used intellectual property law to claim rights

FIG 2.1 / Anthony Atala. From "Growing Body Parts," 60 Minutes, 2009.

over any future inventions using the embryonic stem cell lines it had in its possession. This is what happened with Atala and many other leading regenerative medicine researchers. Geron funded Atala's early research on regenerative medicine in exchange for his signing away his intellectual property rights. The company, Cooper explains, "invented a property right over the uncertain future."[23] By 2014 Geron's only product in development was an experimental therapy for treating myelofibrosis but even that was put on hold by the FDA due to liver risks, causing stock prices to nose-dive and leading one financial journalist to refer to Geron as "a shell company with cash."[24]

Atala testified before the U.S. Senate in 2007 in favor of lifting the Bush administration's ban on federal funding of human embryonic stem cell research. He presented evidence to support his claim that diseases like Parkinson's could be cured within five to ten years if research could move forward without political interference. The military's regenerative medicine programs were not launched until Obama took office and lifted the ban in March 2009, a few months before the 60 Minutes segment aired.[25]

From Atala's laboratory Safer takes us inside the McGowan Institute at the University of Pittsburgh, where we are introduced to Dr. Stephen Badylak, a former veterinarian with degrees in clinical pathology and anatomic pathology. Badylak first began experimenting with cell regeneration in his veterinary practice in 1987, well before tissue engineering was recognized as a field.[26] His initial research subjects were dogs. By the time of the *60 Minutes* segment, he was president of the Tissue Engineering Regenerative Medicine International Society and held over fifty U.S. patents and two hundred patents worldwide. Safer explains how Badylak's laboratory is developing ways to "trick the body into actually repairing and regenerating itself" by using paper-thin connective tissue called the extracellular matrix (ECM) drawn from pig bladders, a substance that is "loaded with signals that instruct cells to do things." ECM is composed from laminin, collagen, and fibronectin, some of the body's largest protein molecules. We learn that, once implanted in the body, ECM eventually breaks down and is replaced by other cells. But first it signals proteins to get to work growing tissue by releasing cryptic peptides that then recruit stem cells to the site of implantation. Pouring some of the powdery substance onto his palm, Badylak teases a reticent Safer, "Want to touch?" Safer demurs and the doctor jokes, "Yes, taking this through airports can be tricky sometimes," an offhand reference to the anthrax scare that occurred several weeks after the events of September 11, in which envelopes filled with a powdery substance were sent by an anonymous source through the U.S. mail, an act of domestic terrorism that turned out to be deadly.[27] The doctor's gallows humor tied biomedical research to the zeitgeist of a Global War on Terror.

In Badylak's laboratory, the pigs' ECM sends a signal communicating the instruction to grow tissue. The bladders are convenient because they are a "throwaway product for the agricultural community" and because "humans have more in common biologically with pigs than they may prefer to believe." Rather than waste the bladders, they are retrieved and stripped of all but the extracellular matrix. Likening the regenerative procedure to a salamander's natural ability to grow a new tail, Badylak explains that humans in the early stages of gestation are able to do the same thing. "If we could make the body or at least part of the body that's missing or injured think that it's an early fetus again, that's game, set, and match." In a subsequent research project, Badylak led a team that used varying electrical currents along with human growth factors, water, and amniotic fluid to build a "bio-

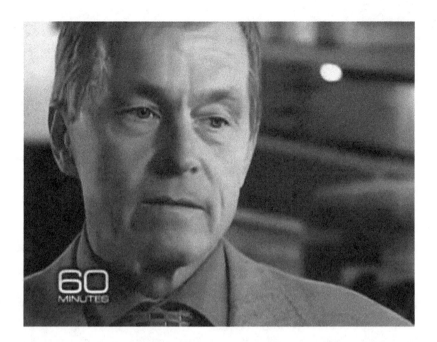

dome" that replicates the conditions of a human embryo. A pair of science journalists summarized the project:

FIG 2.2 / Stephen Badylak. From "Growing Body Parts," 60 *Minutes*, 2009.

"What he is trying to do, in a sense, is make us born again."[28] Biomedical salvation is explained by reference to the spiritual regeneration that is at the heart of Protestant salvationism, in which the human spirit is saved from damnation by being born again.

When Safer and his crew move on to the University of Texas Health Science Center in San Antonio, the focus turns explicitly to military applications of regenerative medicine. We watch six men, each an amputee, sitting on mats in a gym and tossing a ball to one another, as Safer narrates: "The Pentagon has invested $250 million in regenerative research aimed at helping soldiers with severe battle injuries, regrowing muscles and skin for burn injuries as well as transplant technology for lost limbs." Dr. Steven Wolf is the chief of clinical trials at the U.S. Army's Institute for Surgical Research. He is conducting research aimed at stimulating tissue growth in amputee patients by inserting muscle ECM into their bodies where tissue has been lost. Among his patients is Marine Corporal Isais Hernandez, who at the age of nineteen was severely wounded in Afghanistan by a mortar that projected shrapnel into his body. He lost 70 percent of the muscles in

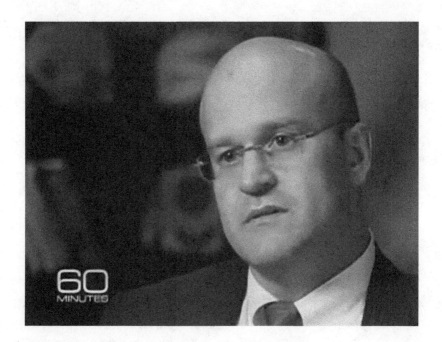

FIG 2.3 / Steven Wolf. From "Growing Body Parts," *60 Minutes*, 2009.

his right thigh. If not for his clutching a 12-inch television he was installing in his convoy truck as part of a makeshift entertainment system for a long road trip, he probably would have died. The TV protected his torso from the onslaught of shrapnel. Doctors told him that the injury to his leg, though, was likely to result in an amputation, which he refused. Hernandez instead asked Wolf, who was one of his doctors, if he could volunteer for a new experimental treatment that the doctor had earlier described as "fertilizing" a wound in order to heal it.[29] In 2008 Wolf's team surgically implanted ECM in Hernandez's thigh in order to stimulate growth; in time the new muscle tissue eventually covered the exposed bone. We watch the young veteran in physical therapy exercising his legs with the guidance of a trainer. "It's remarkable. It's amazing," Safer editorializes as Hernandez speaks about his improved ability to exercise. The trainer adds, "I think there is a lot of potential to see bigger and better things."

Back at the University of Pittsburgh, Marine Corporal Joshua Maloney is a combat engineer and Iraq War veteran who lost a hand during a 2007 training session at Quantico, Virginia, when the explosives he was preparing for a simulation malfunctioned and Maloney was thrown to the

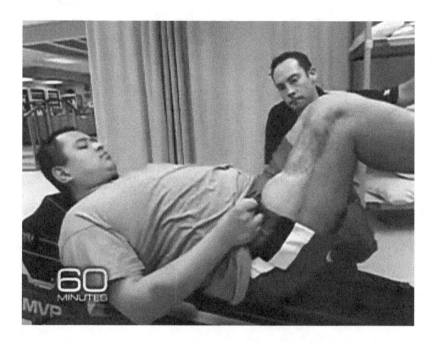

ground. Two years later, in a ten-hour reconstructive surgery, Maloney received a hand transplant from a cadaver. Doctors hoped to avoid admin-

FIG 2.4 / Isais Hernandez with trainer. From "Growing Body Parts," *60 Minutes*, 2009.

istering antirejection drugs and wanted to see if Maloney could rely on his own regenerated cells to attach the hand. What we don't learn from the *60 Minutes* segment is that he ultimately rejected the transplant. The fifty-mile trip from his home to the hospital for regular appointments was wearing him out, and he had to take antirejection drugs to tolerate the transplant. Four years after the surgery, in consultation with his doctors, he reluctantly decided to remove the hand. "I wasn't excited about the decision," he told a Marine Corps journalist. "It felt like I was quitting. It took me a few months and a lot of thinking before I finally reached the decision that we had given it everything we could. It's not working out."[30] As many of the physicians working in this new field acknowledge, much more research is necessary to fulfill the promises of regenerative medicine. They hope to move beyond cultivating small amounts of connective tissue to attach a donor's hand to growing a whole new hand from the patient's own tissue. Innovations also require patients who are willing to participate in certain rehabilitative narratives.[31] For Maloney, the practical matters

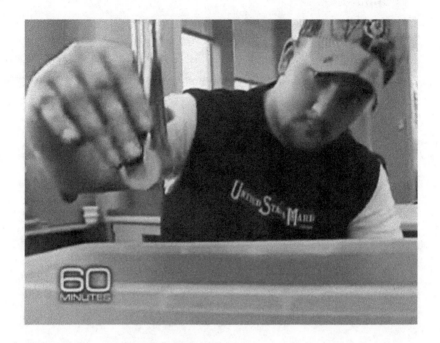

FIG 2.5 / Joshua Maloney. From "Growing Body Parts," 60 *Minutes*, 2009.

of getting to the clinic regularly and participating in a highly experimental course of treatment with adverse effects outweighed the potential miracle that enthused Safer during his tour of regenerative medicine laboratories.

The affable Dr. Wolf reports that his war-injured patients tell him, "Fix me up so I can go back." He is cautious when Safer asks, excitedly, if regenerative medicine works: "It could really change medicine, yes?" It seems to work in terms of regenerating muscle loss but may be more complicated when engineered tissue is placed near a nerve, a bone, or a heart, Wolf qualifies. This doesn't deter the doctor from reiterating the moral urgency that the indebted nation must repay wounded veterans: "These guys, they were protecting us and they took the hit for us and they deserve our respect for that reason. And, from my perspective, they deserve our very best effort to do the best we know how to do and further to do the best that we don't even know yet how to do." These are the last words in the 60 *Minutes* segment: sacrifice and indebtedness, recited in simple terms by a doctor whose knowledge holds the hope of regenerating life.

Here, as in many other popular accounts, the damages wrought by war are registered on the wounded bodies of soldiers to whom a debt is owed.

The researchers, striving to find novel ways of regenerating lost tissue, are key agents of this ever-deferred redemption. They are portrayed in a manner that emphasizes hope, promise, and salvation. Such media stories claim researchers' dedication and skill can atone for the damage not specifically caused by the U.S.-led wars in Afghanistan and Iraq (since the narrative never calls into question the validity or lack thereof of these particular wars) but for war *in the abstract* as signified by the embodied sacrifices of these exemplary veterans struggling to regain ability and be delivered from suffering. They gave their lives to serve the nation, and the nation owes them high-tech healing in return. Redemption is ongoing, not a singular event, in war-related regenerative medicine. It is a biomedical process that has moral dimensions. Its political dimensions, however, are disavowed and therefore become difficult to contest. Miriam Ticktin makes what I consider to be a very useful distinction between "politics" and "the political," specifying that *politics* engages with power and refers to everyday politics, often to policy, "that is, to the set of practices by which *order* is created and maintained." But this is "not *the political*—it is unable to further radical collective change." The political "refers to *the disruption of an established order*."[32] This kind of disruption is disallowed or disavowed within the biomedical salvation narrative that animates the biomedicine-war nexus.

According to this narrative, the nation owes twice for the sacrifices made: once for the wound acquired during the veteran's service to the nation and again for the new technoscientific knowledge that can be derived from the suffering and be of benefit to us all. Redemption of this kind is not achieved in a single payment. Rather the nation's debt reaches into the future. It manifests in forward-looking research proposals, patent applications, and stock portfolios promising regenerated life and profits. Redemption is promised in the form of knowledge production, which is ongoing, like a perpetually hoped-for return on investment. It requires an audience that witnesses and buys the potentially miraculous healing powers of regenerated life, an audience encouraged to have faith in the future as regeneration, an audience asked to recognize the possible life-affirming returns that come in the aftermath of the dreadful investment of waging wars. War wounds, when they leave a signature on the bodies of valorized beings, provide the condition for advancing medical knowledge and building markets. But in order to be regenerated, one must have survived and be capable of learning to be like an early fetus again. Of course we know that many do not survive the lethal consequences of exploding munitions, improvised or otherwise. To be eligible for regeneration, one must count, that is, have value. The regenerated polytraumatized soldier's body is the flag-draped fetal coffin in a fantasy of triumphant war without death.

MILITARY INVESTMENTS IN REGENERATIVE MEDICINE

The U.S. military is so far the biggest investor in the emergent field of regenerative medicine, which was formally recognized by the military when it established the Armed Forces Institute of Regenerative Medicine in 2008. Certain notable features of AFIRM illustrate the complexities of government funding in the context of loosely regulated venture capital investment. President Obama lifted the restrictions on the use of new embryonic stem cells in federally funded research in March 2009. But in the eight years prior to that, as outlined in his Presidential Statement of August 2001, President Bush argued for restricting federal funding for human embryonic stem cell research to the small number of cell lines that had already been cultivated, and funding of new cell lines was banned.[33] On June 20, 2007, Bush signed Executive Order 13435, expanding the approved stem cell lines to be used in "ethically responsible ways": "The Secretary of Health and Human Services shall conduct and support research on the isolation, derivation, production, and testing of stem cells that are capable of producing all or almost all of the cell types of the developing body and may result in improved understanding of or treatments for diseases and other adverse health conditions, but are derived without creating a human embryo for research purposes or destroying, discarding, or subjecting to harm a human embryo or fetus."[34] Obama's Executive Order 13505, signed on March 9, 2009, revoked Bush's Presidential Statement of August 2001 and his Executive Order 13435.

Under Bush's constraints, researchers relied mainly on adult-derived stem cells or turned to private funding sources to support research on embryonic stem cells acquired mostly from fertility clinics whose clients had fulfilled their reproductive goals. During those eight years researchers courted private investors to support stem cell research, emphasizing the likely return on their investments that would come from an expanding new market for regenerative medicine.[35] By 2009, when Obama lifted the ban, a network of industry-paid lobbyists and researchers were happy to learn that the U.S. military, through contracts and grants, would be the largest funder and consumer of regenerative medicine.

Of note in Obama's Executive Order are several passages that reference the promise of regenerative medicine that may someday replace the need for embryonic stem cells by engineering other cells with a similar capacity of pluripotency:

> At this moment, the full promise of stem cell research remains unknown, and it should not be overstated. But scientists believe these tiny cells may have the potential to help us understand, and possibly cure, some of our most devastating diseases and conditions. To regenerate a severed spinal cord and lift someone from a wheelchair. To spur insulin production and spare a child from a lifetime of needles. To treat Parkinson's, cancer, heart disease and others that affect millions of Americans and the people who love them. . . . Ultimately, I cannot guarantee that we will find the treatments and cures we seek. No President can promise that. But I can promise that we will seek them—actively, responsibly, and with the urgency required to make up for lost ground. Not just by opening up this new frontier of research today, but by supporting promising research of all kinds, including groundbreaking work to convert ordinary human cells into ones that resemble embryonic stem cells.[36]

Even with Obama's order lifting the ban on federal funding for stem cell research, business analysts pointed out the high financial risks associated with stem cell research plagued by the "Valley of Death"—the gap in funding that occurs between the time a scientific discovery is made and when the innovation is scaled up in treatments for sale. Venture capitalists were reluctant to invest in a company facing this problem. So university-based scientists and private companies working with stem cells sought state and federal funding to make up for the "moneyless purgatory." Researchers who wouldn't otherwise pitch their research toward military medicine were inclined to do so given the scarcity of other funding sources.[37] For many AFIRM was a magnet.

AFIRM's express purpose was to develop advanced treatment options for severely wounded service members. The Institute facilitated a multi-institutional network and supported collaborative projects involving researchers from the military, academic institutions, and private corporations. The total funding for AFIRM's first five years was around $300 million. Roughly one-third of this was drawn from the army, navy, air force, Veterans Administration, and National Institutes of Health (NIH), another third drawn from matching funds from state governments and participating universities, and a final third from preexisting related research projects funded by NIH, Defense Advanced Research Projects Agency, the National Science Foundation, and private philanthropy.[38] AFIRM was one of seven research concentrations administered through the formidably large U.S. Army Medical Research and Materiel Command (USAMRMC), headquartered at Fort Detrick, Maryland, which also oversaw projects in military infectious diseases, combat casualty care, military operational medicine, clinical and rehabilitative medicine, and medical defense against chemical and biological attacks.

The USAMRMC's wide range of research projects reflected its broad responsibility for medical research and the development of products to be used in military medicine. Laboring under the motto "Protect, Project, and Sustain," some six thousand military, civilian, and contractor personnel were employed by 2011 to support USAMRMC's headquarters and its eleven subordinate commands around the world.[39] The mission of the U.S. Army Telemedicine and Advanced Technology Research Center (TATRC), also part of the USAMRMC, was to explore "high risk and innovative research" with the aim of "putting research findings into the hands of warfighters while looking toward civilian utility."[40] It supported research on health informatics, telemedicine, and computational biology and by 2014 included a special emphasis on advanced prosthetics and neural engineering. Like AFIRM, TATRC was closely tied to the biotechnology industry, drawing together military researchers, university-based scientists, and materials engineers in projects aimed at treating wounded bodies while promising to translate research findings into broader applications, patents, and investment opportunities.

From its early days AFIRM consisted of three main consortia. The first was centered at the U.S. Army Institute of Surgical Research and Brooke Army Medical Center at Fort Sam Houston. Two additional consortia were the Rutgers/Cleveland Clinic Consortium and the Wake Forest Consortium, made up of researchers from leading universities and hospitals around the country, many holding multiple patents on new findings and products they had invented.[41] Each of the two university-based consortia was awarded original seed money from the USAMRMC to cover a five-year period that began in 2007. Each was expected during that time to raise double that amount in additional matching funds to arrive at $80 million, drawing on funding from other public and private sources.

Within its first three years AFIRM had assembled a long list of "industry partners," mainly companies in the biotechnology sector.[42] The exchange of knowledge and resources between military hospitals, university laboratories and research clinics, and for-profit biotechnology corporations was shaped by three key factors: (1) the career-building opportunity to work at the frontiers of regenerative medicine research; (2) the possibility of developing products, devices, and procedures that could be patented and eventually generate profit either through direct sales or speculating on future profits; and (3) the urgency of the perceived problems being addressed (treating polytrauma veterans).

AFIRM researchers engaged in *translational research*, a term of art that emphasizes the movement from laboratory practice to clinical trials in order to deliver goods to patients in a timely fashion, or for what in the past was called applied research. Translational medicine emphasizes efficient movement of research "from bench to bedside" so that laboratory experiments advance to clinical trials and then to point-of-care applications under the pressure of time. The new terminology responds to the pressure not only of current understandings of what the market demands—that science should be aimed at producing products and services ("deliverables") that will yield a profit—but also to the urgency of supporting or saving lives. It represents a trend away from "blue sky" research—also known as "pure research" or "research for knowledge's sake alone"—because this kind of knowledge, especially when it is paid for by taxpayers, is seen to be too slow and potentially wasteful. University-based researchers labor under conditions that subject them to institutional demands to raise money through grant applications or capital investment in order to keep their laboratories operating. The temptations are great for choosing to do research that is more likely to get grants and attract investors and result in products that later trade well on the stock market. Though investing in biotechnology is speculative and risky, its appeal lies in its claim to bring spectacular future returns. Regenerative medicine draws on the fantasy of perpetual generation not only in producing tissue and cures but also in yielding profit.

ANTICIPATING NEEDS AND (RE)GENERATING FUTURES

Biotechnology is anticipatory, generating new markets and responding to projected future needs. Regenerative medicine, understood within this framing, is a form of promissory capital that counts on the hope and hype of generative futures. It is one of many "futures generators" in regimes of anticipation.[43] Regenerative medicine operates within a metaphysics of renewal resonant with technoscientific salvation, tacking back and forth between futures, pasts, and presents. It shuttles between the condition of loss to a past before the damage occurred and then to a future when cells will regenerate new tissue. In the parlance of regenerative medicine researchers, the body must learn to be like a fetus again in order to move into the future.

As shown in the *60 Minutes* segment and the military's projected hopes in treating war-related polytrauma veterans, regenerative medicine brings together stem cell science and tissue engineering. Regenerative medicine is conceptualized as a second-generation model of earlier biomedical technologies such as prosthetics and organ transplantation, sharing an interest in repairing or enhancing bodily function.[44] The history of tissue engineering dates from the early 1990s, when stem cell biology emerged as an important innovation. By the late 1990s at laboratories in the United States, Europe, and South Korea, scientists working in this field had achieved the culturing of pluripotent human embryonic stem cell lines and discovered that adult stem cells were more ubiquitous and plastic than had been assumed.

Tissue engineering seeks to reconstruct three-dimensional living organs and tissues in vitro, from the cellular level up before they are transplanted into the patient's body. It differs from reconstructive medicine because it doesn't simply transfer tissues through microsurgery techniques; it also seeks to modulate the morphogenesis of these tissues, in vitro and in vivo. It is concerned with the genesis of form rather than the transplantation of already given forms. The field is a stronger descendant of experimental embryology than it is of the fields of prosthetics and organ transplantation. It is, in other words, more concerned with self-assembly through the pluripotency of embryonic or progenitor cells. Like embryology, regenerative medicine does not suspend animation and then replace a limb or organ but instead intervenes in the process of morphogenesis to modulate or redirect this process. As Cooper notes, rather than requiring the organ to be frozen, tissue engineering works with and exploits the active responsiveness of living tissue and its ability to change in time, under the conditions of varying kinds of forces (biochemical, mechanical, hydrodynamic, and electromagnetic) and operating in relation to which various qualities (density, compressibility, and elasticity).[45]

Sources of tissue used in engineering projects include living cells from aborted fetuses, umbilical cords, and frozen embryos—products of female bodies—as well as the discarded foreskins of circumcised male children and, more recently, urine. Tissue engineering makes use of autologous (self-to-self) cloning of cells from one region of a patient's body to be cultivated in another region (similar to skin grafting for burn victims). Encompassed in this horizon of therapeutic cloning is the practice of gathering autologous embryonic tissue to clone cells that may be used later in one's life in the event of tissue injury (such as burns or spinal cord trauma), chronic illness (such as diabetes), or cellular degeneration (such as amyotrophic lateral sclerosis or Alzheimer's disease). The industry of stem cell banking allows clients to deposit cells that can be used later to reconstitute the immune system after chemotherapy, for example, or to generate nerve cell tissues to treat Parkinson's disease. But tissue banking is expensive and not yet proven to be effective over the long term. Even so, by 2008 companies with names like StemLifeLine, Cryo-Cell International, Neo-Stem, MediStem Laboratories, and C'elle charged fees for collecting and processing cells that ranged from $499 to $7,500, depending on the company, and between $89 and $699 annually for storing the cells in liquid nitrogen. They collected cells from an expanding number of sources, including menstrual fluid, baby's teeth, and even fat removed by liposuction.

Scientists disagree about the efficacy of stem cell banking. Those with direct and indirect financial interests in the industry argue for its value. Others working independently at laboratories and clinics, who are not shareholders in cell banking companies, tend to be more skeptical about the enterprise. In a 2008 interview with the *New York Times*, Christopher Scott, Stanford University's director of the Program on Stem Cells in Society, warned, "In the stem cell area, we have a problem of truth in advertising. Some of these companies are skirting right on the edge of what's truthful and what's vaporware."[46] A company called BioEden Inc., based in Austin, Texas, promised, "One day, the Tooth Fairy could save your child's life," suggesting that the stem cells contained in baby teeth could be cultivated to grow many different kinds of cells. BioEden reported having a thousand customers in 2009. Each was charged $595 per tooth extraction and an annual fee of $89 for storing the cultivated cells. The company sought out teeth from dentists and elementary schools, offering to pay $100 per tooth. BioEden's claims were overstated in the view of Pamela Gehron Robey, who headed the NIH laboratory that discovered baby-teeth stem cells. "There's never been a demonstration that these cells actually form nerve cells that can function as nerve cells," she told a reporter for the *New York Times*.[47] The American Academy of Pediatrics issued a policy statement in January 2007 warning against the private banking of umbilical cord blood as "biological insurance" for children without a known risk for disease.

The hope of tissue engineers is to develop techniques and products that can overcome the problems that commonly occur with organ transplantation and prosthetics: immune reactions, the scarcity and fragility of transplantable organs, and the limited life span of medical implants in the body that break down from wear and tear. Tissue engineering works with the regenerative capacities of the body so that once the substituted cells are placed in the body (having been cultured in vitro), the body's processes would regenerate an organ or tissue, eliminating the problem of immune-related rejections. When explaining this process to lay audiences, stem cell researchers often say that all mammalian fetuses have the capacity to regenerate limbs in utero and that human children under the age of four are able to regrow lost fingertips, a capacity that wanes with aging. Exploiting the regenerative and pluripotent capabilities of embryonic stem cells is narrativized as a recapturing of youth—going backward in the interests of futurity.

One line of regenerative medicine research involves burn victims. Invasive and painful skin graft procedures are replaced by a technique called "cell spraying" that "takes a postage stamp sized piece of a burn victim's healthy skin, exposing it to an enzyme that separates the cells from each other, and then immediately spraying them onto the damaged skin."[48] In one case reported by AFIRM, a burn victim received fat cells injected under the burn scars in order to restore flexibility and movement (also known as "scarless wound healing"). In another research project aimed at developing a regenerative bandage for battlefield wounds, a Stanford team sought to use a biomimetic matrix and human progenitor cells to prevent the onset of scarring, fibrosis, and infection. By inducing a "pro-regenerative state of suspended animation," the researchers hoped to re-create a "fetal-like wound healing milieu" to promote regeneration immediately after the wound occurs and to restore function so that a wounded soldier may return to fight.[49] The imagery of a fetal healing milieu seems like a salve to ease the physical and psychological vulnerability caused by what was added more recently to the list of signature injuries associated with the recent wars in

Iraq and Afghanistan: genital injuries suffered by previously able-bodied men and described by physicians and soldiers alike as inflicting a fate worse than death.[50] But what would it take to trick their wounded bodies into thinking they are early fetuses again? A first step involved rabbits.

SCENARIO: REGENERATION AND REALITY

Prior to his work with AFIRM, Dr. Atala had long been interested in developing treatments for genital injuries caused by work- and sports-related accidents, vehicle collisions, and other traumatic events. When urogenital casualties surged among American troops, he wanted to help them by bringing his expertise in urology into the field of regenerative medicine. In November 2009 his team reported the successful regeneration of the castrated penises of twelve New Zealand white rabbits, using the same techniques they had used to regenerate a pig's bladder.[51] Like bladders, penises require a cavernous structure to allow for expansion and contraction, so Atala's success with bladder regenesis offered a promising chance for penile tissue regeneration. The experiment began with castrating a group of twenty-seven rabbits. Researchers retained the castrated penises in order to compare them later with the tissue they would regenerate, specifically in terms of comparing the amount of pressure in the *caverna* of the original penises with that of the newly grown penile tissue toward the goal of achieving erection. The endothelial cells that line the blood vessels and smooth muscle cells were harvested from the penile tissue of the rabbits. These were multiplied in vitro and then injected, over a two-day period, into a collagen scaffolding to provide support as they grew. The multistep "cell-seeding" injections allowed the scaffolds to hold many more smooth muscle cells than in previous studies involving muscle tissue. This in turn allowed for the flexibility required for achieving an erection, in which the endothelial cells release nitric oxide, thus triggering smooth muscle relaxation and an influx of blood.

Once the scaffolds seemed ready, they were implanted in twenty-four of the rabbits. Twelve were implanted with matrices that were seeded with cells. Twelve others were implanted with unseeded scaffolding, constituting a positive control group. The remaining three castrated rabbits received no replacement cells or scaffolding in order to function as a negative control group. Within a month the implanted tissue, including smooth muscle and blood vessels, began to form in the twelve who received seeded scaffolds. Once the experimental rabbits healed, each was placed in a cage with a female rabbit, first at one month into the research, then at three months, and finally at six months. Each of the rabbits with seeded scaffolds (i.e., working penile tissue) attempted copulation within a minute of exposure to their female partners at each interval. Four of those females were impregnated, and eight showed the presence of sperm. Most of the males with only scaffolding but no working tissue did not attempt copulation, and none showed the presence of sperm. The three negative control rabbits simply did not attempt to mate with female partners. The most important breakthrough achieved in this study was the regeneration of what is known as the *corpora cavernosa penis*, the erectile tissue of the penis, whose virtue is the ability to fill with blood during an erection. In a press release announcing the study's findings, Atala remarked, "These results are encouraging. They indicate the possibility of using laboratory-engineered tissue in men who require reconstructive procedures. A lack of erectile tissue currently prevents us from restoring sexual function to these patients."[52]

Science journalists reported that Atala's findings offered hope to wounded male veterans who faced psychological barriers to treatment. Many of the injured were reluctant to follow up on referrals to specialists performing phalloplasty, in which doctors use skin grafts to build an artificial penis. "I ain't going to no sex-change doctor," said one injured marine. Referring to a photo he had seen of penises constructed from surgical flaps taken from patients' arms, he told a journalist, "I could do better with Silly Putty."[53] A penis regenerated by tissue engineering that might allow a man to experience sensation, to achieve an erection, and to have his fertility restored seemed far more appealing than phallopasty.

Despite its encouraging results in rabbits, Atala's tissue engineering could not remedy the wide range of sexual dysfunction resulting from blast wounds suffered by veterans. In some patients exposure to blasts caused testosterone levels and sperm counts to fall, even among those who experienced no direct injury to the genitals. Some patients were given testosterone to increase sex drive and restore energy, but many suffering from blast injuries were also on a cocktail of antiswelling and antipain drugs that canceled or mitigated the intended effects of testosterone replacement. Posttraumatic psychological stress and some of the medications to treat it have a depressing effect on libido. Regenerating penile tissue, thus considered, is only one of the many treatments that are necessary to restore sexual and reproductive function in many injured veterans.

Masculine prowess is valorized in U.S. Army Infantry and Marine Corps culture, branches of service where war-related genital injuries were most common. Though seldom discussed in media stories or included in regenerative medicine clinical trials, women soldiers and marines sustained these injuries too, requiring in some cases reconstructive surgery and, when ovaries were destroyed, hormone replacement therapy. Most media accounts described men's injuries as particularly psychologically devastating to the veteran's identity and hope for the future. For example, journalist David Wood interviewed a group of patients, including a twenty-three-year-old who served as a rifleman in the Marine Corps. Mark Litynski had been married for about a year when he received orders that he would be deployed. "I ought to freeze my sperm so we could still have kids if something happened," he recalled thinking. But he never got around to it by the time he left for Afghanistan in September 2010. Two months later, while on combat patrol, an IED exploded near him; he lost both his legs and most of his left arm, his pelvis was shattered, and debris penetrated his abdominal cavity. The blast severely damaged his genitals. Injured men like Corporal Litynski were left, in Wood's words, "unable to father children and struggling to engage in something resembling the sex they used to have, often without the aid of what many view as the primary symbol of their manhood."[54]

Speaking with patients and medical specialists at Walter Reed, Wood discovered a severe shortage of properly trained specialists to treat these injuries effectively. Available treatments were physically agonizing and cost more than insurance would cover. Patients complained of not getting the psychological help they needed to deal with such a devastating loss. The miracles promised by regenerative medicine were a far cry from addressing the basic needs and hopes for the future of these patients. For Wood, the young marines' infertility and the sacrifice it signified underscored the debt that is owed to them by the nation they served.

The anthropologist Zoë H. Wool provides a poignant account of the experiences of severely wounded soldiers going through the complex process of rehabilitation and the entanglements of this process with intimacy, sexuality, and identity. Wool spent many hours with patients, their lovers, and their families at Walter Reed in 2007 and 2008. Her analysis brings to light how the icon of the soldier's body as a national symbol of normative masculinity was unsettled by the physically and emotionally taxing nature of their treatment regimes. "The all-too-common narrative," she writes, "of the heroic wounded veteran as the embodiment of patriotic self-sacrifice" is disrupted by the experience of severe injury and painstaking rehabilitation. Patients require care and contact with and from their loved ones, their caregivers, and each other. Their ontological status is rooted in these tender biosocial relations. Wool observed the contradictory character of U.S. heteronational ideals of independence experienced by the male soldier-patients: on the one hand was the ideal of the independent individual in charge of his own body and not dependent upon others (i.e., not disabled and therefore not "less human"), and on the other hand was the valorization of a particular kind of dependency manifesting in the heterosexual conjugal couple, where personhood and life are expected to be "secured for the future."[55]

Examining this contradiction Wool theorized intimacy as an embodied political relation between those bodies "whose animating force is the field of sexuality."[56] Self-sufficiency was a goal of rehabilitation but was achievable only through a sustained dependency upon significant others. Intimate attachments in heterosexual conjugal couplehood, as difficult as they may have been to enact, were "lifelines" among this patient population unique in its intimate familiarity with both killing and dying. Death seemed proximate, looming, and anticipated in those patients who kept to themselves, withdrawing from loved ones. Being alone was dangerous. But intimacy and connection, while necessary, were fraught. Biological life is never solitary or isolated; it requires attachments. Though a condition of life generally, these attachments were acutely experienced by the injured men Wool encountered.

Drawing on Beth Linker's work, Wool contrasts the ideology of rehabilitation that followed World War I with that of the post-9/11 era, noting that the former focused on masculinizing, self-sufficiency, and independence as goals of rehabilitation that were reflective of ideals of productive ablebodiedness and inflected with ideas about racial hygiene consonant with the far-flung eugenics movement of the time.[57] By contrast, in the post-9/11 era the properly functioning heterosexual conjugal couple is exalted as the goal and privileged signifier of successful rehabilitation. The ties that bind this couple are not exclusively sexual but entail what Wool calls "a properly intimate attachment between two bodies." Bodies of the conjugal couple must be gendered in proper ways; they must perform and be iterative according to a dyadic framework dividing masculinity from femininity. But under the circumstances of grave injury, bodies require so much care and touch and attention that properly intimate requirements of conjugal couplehood are often obstructed or foreclosed. Masculinity, as symbolized by erection, penetration, and ejaculation, is perilous and precarious. Wool found that masculinity among soldier-patients was "most securely refashioned not through the work of or on a body alone *but through the attachments and forms of touch that make up the conjugal couple.*"[58] The high rates of prescribed erectile dysfunction drugs for young married soldiers at Walter Reed indicated an awareness on the part of physicians of the value invested in restoring heterosexual masculine sexual embodiment, a value often shared by patients themselves, intimate partners, and therapists. Normative forms of reproductive masculinity therefore entailed a drug-dependent prosthetic masculinity that was to be tied to matrimonial sexuality aimed at restoring pleasure and generating reproductive futures. But, as Wool observes, the conjugal couple existed within a web of other intimacies, foremost among them the ties that bind men who have served together in war, since, as is often recited by veterans, no one but those who went through the experience of fighting wars can possibly understand what they have been through or continue to be going through. Even among noninjured soldiers, the heterosexual conjugal couple and the children they produce are often in tension with the homosocial fraternity of interconnectedness and dependency on others in one's unit. There is, in other words, a complex tension between autological selfhood and collective affiliation. This is exacerbated under the circumstances of grave injury.

While the hyperbolic promotion of heterosexual masculinity provides ideological cover for the homosocial and homoerotic attachments that compose military culture, not all soldiers suffering from genital wounds or sexual dysfunction were heterosexual or male. The reality of losing one's ability to experience sexual pleasure is significant no matter what one's sexual orientation or gender identity. Some attachments are severed by the experience of wounding, others forged because of it. Polytrauma is always emotional and psychosexual, whether it is the leg, the arm, the brain, or the genitalia that are wounded. Sexual functioning encompasses much more than the ability to procreate. It deeply defines the self and the self's relation to others. But little media attention has been paid to soldier-patients suffering from genital injuries outside the framework of conjugal couplehood and heteronormative reproductive imperatives. In these narratives, getting the body to "think like a fetus again" occupies a chimerical relationship to getting hard and getting off for the sake of having a future. Permanent embryogenesis and prosthetic erectile function are promissory elements in this narrative of heteronationalist salvation. The significance of the injury is linked in these accounts to ideologies of sexuality and gender and race that obscure many other damaging facets of war attachments, valorizing reproductive patriotism and eschewing nonnormative lives and bodies of compatriots as well as those belonging to the enemy.

SYNOPSIS

This chapter centered on polytrauma, a devastating injury resulting from the confluence of proliferating explosive devices, greater protective gear, and advancements in evacuation and emergency medicine. Polytrauma indexes a woundscape brought into being by the complex provocations among weaponry, tactics, and medical procedures within a specific geopolitical history of American empire. A vulnerological analysis of the injury's diagnosis and proposed treatments reveals the technofuturistic hopes that attach to suffering. It also exposes the asymmetrical relationship between combatants. One set of combatants in the conflict has enormous technological capacity to conduct war by using air power, well-trained forces, advanced weaponry, sophisticated surveillance technology, and efficient emergency field medicine, but this group can be severely disabled by the improvisations of its opponent, a smaller and less well equipped group that salvages ordnance and builds handmade bombs capable of severe bodily devastation.

The bodies of the more powerful force that survive are among those enlisted to participate in experimental treatments that anticipate a future of regenerated life. Regenerative medicine counts on survivors of injuries for its interventions and advancements to biomedicine. Those who do not survive do not count. Neither do those whose deaths and injuries are not encompassed in the narrative of regenerative medicine's promises. This includes not only enemy combatants but also many who are caught in the crossfire of this asymmetrical warfare. It also includes war-wounded American troops who question the efficacy of treatment or give up on it altogether.

I have argued that the condition of war-related polytrauma, when experienced by U.S. veterans, is a central element in popular accounts of the promises offered by regenerative medicine. In this new horizon of biomedical research, the bodies of the significantly injured patients—primarily

American soldiers and marines—signify a double indebtedness that entangles war with medicine and enlists ordinary citizens to acknowledge this debt and repay it in a variety of affective and material ways. An abstract formation—the nation—owes twice for the sacrifices made: once for the wound acquired when the warrior served the nation and again for the new technoscientific knowledge that can be derived from medical treatment of the warrior's suffering. This, I have argued, is one way technoscientific and biomedical promises provide a means through which attachments to war manifest.

The condition of indebtedness, understood in the imaginary of regenerative medicine, is tied up with a process of salvation that, rather than settling a debt, reaches into the future. It comes in the form of ongoing knowledge production figured around the promising regeneration of life ad infinitum. Salvaging life through technoscience is a perpetual process that regenerates life and promises a return on (affective and financial) investment. And the jarring reality is that this horizon of research stands in stark contrast to the simultaneous conditions under which particular lives—understood as complex social processes injured by geopolitical economic forces—are permanently disabled as an effect of surviving horrific attacks.

I have also argued that rehabilitative treatment regimes and regenerative tissue engineering are tied to heteronormative and heteronationalist ideological formations within the contexts encountered in this chapter. Restoring, repaying, and regenerating severely injured male soldiers' bodies are interwoven processes that evince a cultural anxiety about the fragility of American masculinity and what it takes to maintain it. In scenarios where fragile, anxious, or doubtful biosocial attachments reside alongside an epidemic of suicide, hopeful investment in biomedicine signifies a sentiment of care and a gesture of ongoing perilous redemption. In narratives of polytrauma, regeneration, rehabilitation, and reproduction are interwoven aspirations that draw together investments in patriotic heterosexual masculinity that, as I have been arguing, attach biomedicine to war through sentiments of hope and dramas of salvation.

In approaching the crisis of war-related polytrauma and the promises it poses for biotechnological futures, I am not arguing against scientific research. Instead I am arguing for seeing it as implicated in moral and political economies in which value is measured by speculation in an imaginary future and in which biotechnology is presented as capable of generating ever-returning gains. This future, I believe, is in contrast to the realities of injury, despair, and death faced by many who are severely injured in war and who lack meaningful access to health care. While regenerative medicine is promoted as a potential miracle treatment, it is certainly not mentioned as a suitable treatment for any of the tens of thousands of severely wounded Iraqis and Afghans, including women and children. They remain invisible and uncared for. They are, in a biopolitical sense, abandoned.

THREE

We Can Enhance You

On Bionic Prosthetics

During a 2006 interview on *NewsHour*, the nightly program aired by the Public Broadcasting System, a young, energetic artist and bionics engineer responded to the interviewer's question about working with the Defense Advanced Research Projects Agency (DARPA). David Hanson wanted to help wounded U.S. troops whose faces were destroyed in severe blast explosions:

> I thought that we are in a time of great convergence and that we could solve a great deal of human suffering if we could push the revolutions of biotechnology and tissue engineering and robotics together—to better administer to wounded soldiers and civilians as well. There are many more civilians with these kinds of injuries actually in the world and they'll benefit from this convergence of technology. [If] we can create these technologies to address our combat injuries, then we can alleviate so much misery in the world. I felt absolutely confident that a revolution in medicine was going to result from the conversations that were taking place at that event.[1]

Hugh Herr, an engineer and biophysicist at the MIT Media Lab, is at the cutting edge of research on bionic devices designed for amputees.[2] Recognized for his contributions to human rehabilitation, Herr remarked in a 2014 interview, "The war on terrorism has unleashed a tremendous amount of funding for this area. If you plot innovation in prosthetics over time, spikes of activity always occur after war."[3] A caption next to a photograph of Herr in his lab, included in a 2008 *Christian Science Monitor* article, reads, "Hugh Herr says he had trouble finding funding for his research into prosthetic limbs before U.S. forces invaded Iraq. Now, thanks to military grants, his innovations can help both soldiers and civilians. . . . Throughout history, war has presented unique challenges that have spurred and inspired the development of new technologies—inventions that may have taken years, or even decades, to evolve in the civilian market. After more than five years, the wars in Iraq and Afghanistan have begun to leave their footprint on science history."[4]

In 2008 U.S. Army Colonel (retired) Geoff Ling, a neurological physician and founding director of the DARPA Biological Technologies Office, spoke with reporters about his office's Revolutionizing Prosthetics program, then in its second year: "Amputees everywhere in the country and possibly the world are going to benefit from this. . . . Out of the tragedy of war comes an opportunity for a lot of people."[5]

———————

I begin with these three snapshots, each featuring an expert in prosthetics engineering. They personify connections between biomedical research and war. As wounded troops returned from the wars in Iraq and Afghanistan, researchers working on neural bionics turned their attention to this growing population of patients. War provided them with an opportunity to accelerate their research. And in the midst of this acceleration, publicity about this growing field emphasized its value for rehabilitating veterans' bodies. But even more was at stake, the researchers argued. The knowledge they were developing and the devices they were designing had the potential to augment the human body. In their technophilic narrative, all bodies would someday have the potential to be superhuman. Fantasies of superseding the limits of human embodiment were woven into the fabric of media depictions that centered on the injured bodies of returning warriors. Biomedical salvationism was at the heart of these depictions. Supporting new research initiatives was articulated as a way to honor those who sacrificed their lives for the nation. A promise to alleviate their suffering was coupled with grandiose dreams of augmenting life.

Focusing on bionic prosthetics design, in this chapter I explore some of the complex material and psychological attachments to war through another example in which injuries stimulate new products and new knowledge. Cutting-edge prosthetic devices literalize attachments to war for those fitted with them. They also serve as haunting reminders of the damage war causes for those bearing witness to their promised capabilities.

Bionic assemblages, as they were featured in media stories, link the domains of fitness culture, "x-treme sports," and performance art to artificial intelligence and computational robotics through their charismatic designers. Normative assumptions about gender, sexuality, beauty, ability, and intelligence are embedded in bionic devices, drawing audiences into dramatic encounters with bodies whose injuries signify the effects of living in a dangerous world and who, in rehabilitative regimes of vigilant resilience, come to stand for the cherished ideological tenets of freedom, liberty, and national belonging.

Considerable money is involved in this turn toward cybernetic prosthetics research. By 2014 the U.S. military had become a major funding source for this field. University-based researchers, many of whom owned start-up companies, teamed up with military physicians in a manner similar to the situation in regenerative medicine. In the circuitry of federal funding, ordinary citizens were attached to this research through the taxes they paid. But more than that, a tech-curious public was invited to witness the miracles of new prosthetic designs in TED Talks, *Wired* magazine articles, and YouTube demonstrations. Scientists, physicians, engineers, and artists working in prosthetics propose a form of vital materialism that involves technoscientific salvation coupled with an aesthetic of enhancement. The vitality of bionics extended beyond their simulations of natural functions; it depended substantially on the publicly witnessed performance of patients' dedication to improving their conditions. By the second decade of the twenty-first century, the hard work of veterans recovering from war-related disfigurement was central to the enterprise and appeal of body-enhancement technologies.

Beginning around 2005 inventors Hanson and Herr spoke of their new prosthetic devices as a means by which to repay the nation's debt to injured soldiers. They promised that bionic prosthetics would restore bodily capabilities while making warfare more efficient and, paradoxically, life-affirming. Damaged bodies, if successfully rebuilt, would recast war as a source of vitality rather than of death and destruction. But for miracles to emerge, severely injured bodies were required. Something and someone needed to be salvageable. Claims of beneficence and care, central to the biomedical logics I outlined in previous chapters, infused the discourses offered by Hanson, Herr, Ling, and other bionics researchers funded by DARPA. In addition to inventing artificial faces, legs, arms, and hands, some were busy producing robots they described as compassionate and experimenting with neural systems they hoped would advance scientific knowledge about the workings of the human brain and the nervous system in general. The beneficiaries would not be just the injured patients but extended to *everyone*—a code word for members of the American public. Promissory logics were evident in these inventors' discourse, where bionic innovations were not simply regarded as substitutions for missing or damaged body parts but seen as superior to nature's design. In their technoscientific vision, bodies were biotechnologies to be modified, engineered, and improved but not without the genius minds that were able to work this magic.

THE ENCHANTMENTS OF ENHANCEMENT

During the first decades of the twenty-first century, popular and medical journalism presented innovations in bionics and prosthetics engineering as hopeful responses to the growing number of war-related polytrauma patients. The U.S. military reported that, between 2001 and the end of 2013, the total number of major limb amputation patients resulting from battle injuries was 1,558 for active-duty men and women serving in Iraq and Afghanistan.[6] Media coverage of bionics involving wounded veterans typically represented this field of research in miraculous terms, cultivating a quality of enchantment with technology that, when compared with the practical results, resonates with Berlant's notion of cruel optimism. The double bind, here, "in which your attachment to an object sustains you in life at the same time as that object is actually a threat to your flourishing," will be evident in some of the specific research projects and the stories of patients hoping that what they had lost could be restored.[7] But first it helps to provide a description of the field of bionics research as it relates to biomedical logics.

When used in medicine, *bionics* generally refers to the replacement or enhancement of body parts or organs with mechanical versions that mimic original natural functions. It shares some meaning with the terms *biomimicry* and *biomimetics*, both coined in the 1950s to designate the emerging science using knowledge derived from biology about natural systems to apply to the design of engineering systems, notably sonar, radar, and cochlear implants. The term was made popular by the 1970s weekly television dramas *The Six Million Dollar Man* and *The Bionic Woman*, which centered on main characters whose bodies were rebuilt after sustaining severe accidents. With the aid of bionic implants they gained superhuman powers.

Computer-driven bionic devices are reflective of a specific historical and cultural context in which the body is imagined to have ever-expanding potential. The bodies of severely wounded veterans of recent wars—those who would not have survived under previous conditions—are central to bionic narratives of the future enhancement and expanded potential of human bodies. These patients' significant injuries, as I outlined in chapter 2, afford the inventors of bionic prosthetics opportunities to demonstrate the salvific power of technoscientific innovations. They present artfully orchestrated performances to audiences sympathetic to injured veterans but also eager to learn how these new devices may enhance their own lives. By witnessing what could be done to restore amputees' otherwise lost abilities, audiences of TED Talks and television shows like *60 Minutes* were invited to look forward to a future when bioengineering would enable humanity to surpass a host of bodily limitations.

Innovations in bionic prosthetics reflect a broader cultural investment in the idea of fashioning the body as a way to fulfill the self, using various technologies to make bodies better. "Better" here is a hegemonic formulation organized around normative standards of productivity, visual appeal, and physical acumen. Increased longevity and even immortality are part of the biotechnological fantasy of extending the capabilities of bodies. In recent decades the market has been flooded with consumer-grade enhancement devices and products. Among these are anabolic steroids for enhancing stamina and athletic performance, pharmacological drugs to enhance memory and concentration, hormones to slow down the effects of aging, drugs that purport to stimulate libido by enabling erectile function, beta blockers to overcome stage fright, and human growth hormone for increasing the height of smaller than average children. Enhancement technologies also include elective cosmetic surgery as well as procedures in reproductive medicine aimed at producing babies with what parents and doctors take to be desirable characteristics. Software products and microprocessors are also enhancement technologies. For example, a proliferating number of apps for smartphones supplement their users' memory. They can enhance users' awareness of their physical fitness and diet, their consciousness about levels of stress and anxiety, and their sense of navigational direction. Apple's voice simulator, Siri, uses basic artificial intelligence to respond to and serve the user. All of these enhancement products are encompassed in an expanded definition of *prosthetic*, which has a dual meaning, standing for a replacement or substitute as well as an addition, augmentation, or enhancement.

The term *prosthetic* has animated much critical theorizing about the relationship between bodies and technologies in science and technology studies and in disability studies. One tendency has manifested in appropriating the term as a central metaphor for analyzing postmodern cultural processes, politics, and aesthetics.[8] Marquard Smith and Joanne Morra critically engage what they call "the prosthetic impulse," admitting their reluctance about this generalizing gesture because "the prosthetic" has assumed an epic status in technoscience studies, cinema studies, speculative fiction, artificial intelligence, virtual reality, and postmodern warfare that is "out of proportion with its abilities to fulfill our ambitions for it." At the same time the authors seek to explore the metaphorical potential of prosthesis for speculation, analysis, and interpretation, looking at the connections between the metaphorical and material connotations of the term. They interrogate the "metaphorical optimism" of the prosthetic imagination in order to "reassert the phenomenological, material, and *embodied* nature of the prosthetic impulse."[9] My own approach is aligned with critical interventions from the field of disability studies that emphasize the historically situated and specific materiality of prosthetics science, its practitioners, its patient populations, and its products.[10] Eschewing a technofetishistic tendency, I am interested instead in the material conditions under which certain bodies are targeted for correction or enhancement. The wounded veteran's body is mobilized in the fantasies of enhancement in ways I will detail shortly.

Consumer capitalism is a significant force for selling the idea of enhancement to a wide audience, manufacturing needs and new identities through the goods and services that individuals believe may make up for their bodies' shortcomings. Endorsements of expert-guided fitness routines, "mental wellness" programs, and dietary regimes flood human resources department brochures, Internet screens, newsstands, reality television shows, and infomercials, promising ways to overcome limitations and past traumas and become new and improved versions of ourselves. Makeover culture traffics in an imaginary of redemptive enhancement that puts a premium on the visual, the stock and trade of commercial advertising: if you look better, you will feel better. Aesthetic evaluations matter very much in this realm. This is brought to the fore in treating war-related disfigurement. Doctors and engineers are likened to artists sculpting materials into beautiful form out of the ravages of severe injury.

Market pressures increase the range of possible capabilities to be enhanced or improved upon. Cultural values of self-making, productivity, and flexibility are reflected in enhancement fantasies. Tropes of personal mastery, empowerment, self-esteem, and adaptability run through prescriptions for living a responsible life in twenty-first-century America. In this ideological framework poverty is regarded as a sign of moral failure. So is what is perceived to be an unwillingness to challenge the body's limitations or flaws. For all persons—but in particular ways for disabled persons—the future invades the present not only in terms of anticipating risks and dangers but also in terms of hoping for better days ahead, achieved through a technoscientific form of "faith healing," having faith in technology and in working hard, being resilient, striving for improvement, and treating misfortune as an opportunity to become a better self. Hopefulness and appropriate willfulness are crucial affective dispositions woven into the discourses about prosthetics. But to whom are these forms of hope, faith, and willpower available? How much does it cost to work on the self? Who can effectively exercise the duty to be healthy? Who is discounted in the regime of self-improvement? In the economy of war-related biomedicalization, select injured veterans undertaking rehabilitation become exemplars of the politics of hope and hard work. Their achievements are commonly narrated in terms of rehabilitation and also in the futuristic terms of robobionic superiority. But rehabilitation and expensive bionic devices are not available to the injured whose bodies and lives are not counted—those who are relegated to what the disability studies scholar H. M. Lukes calls hypohabilitation.[11]

SORTING THE WORTHY FROM THE UNWORTHY

People who suffer disabling conditions and then dedicate great effort to overcoming them by making use of scientific knowledge and technology hold a special place in the moral economy of twenty-first-century self-making. Accounts of their rehabilitation become parables about the virtues of perseverance. The dominant rehabilitative bionics narrative valorizes once vital individuals who suffer an injury that sets them back and from which they strive to recover. They are subjects of hyperhabilitation, a process available to people regarded as worth caring for because of who (or what cause) they have served, what they have lost, and the hope that they inspire. According to this moral evaluation, the veteran's war-injured body (typically depicted as young, white, and male) is at the top of the value hierarchy, having sacrificed his vitality for the greater good of the nation and then submitted to the rigors of expert-guided and technologically sophisticated rehabilitation. A similarly valorized person is the paralympic athlete, who dedicates great effort to competing in sports activities. The veteran who competes as a paralympian is the quintessential figure of hyperhabilitation. By contrast, subjects of hypohabilitation are deemed not worthy of care either because they are blamed for their disabilities or, it is assumed, they have nothing to lose. Among them are grouped together people who were severely disabled from birth or who lack the resources to follow through on rehabilitation following an injury. Into this latter category are disabled persons in impoverished communities, persons with disabilities that cause them to behave counter to social norms, and people belonging to a nation or group with which we are at war. Subjects of hypohabilitation are abandoned in the framework of enhancement.

David Serlin notes a distinction between "the 'tragically' disabled and the congenitally 'deformed'" in his analysis of how disabled veterans have been valued above others. Because veterans' disabilities are induced by modern technology and war, they signify a commitment to the modern state, to industrial capitalism, and to warfare. The veteran's body exemplifies patriotic values and valorizes masculinity, and when it is damaged, the nation owes a debt to its rehabilitation. Disabilities induced by heredity factors or illnesses occupy a lower status, casting "deformed" bodies as incompetent and a drain on society, "inimical to patriotic value or normative manly competence and productivity."[12]

But, as Rosemary Garland-Thomson argues, ambivalence surrounds disability in modern American society. On the one hand, we have legal instruments such as the Americans with Disabilities Act of 1990 that are intended to protect against discrimination and to mandate the public accommodation of disabled persons. On the other hand, Americans tend to assume that eliminating a disability would be better than accommodating it. The nation's troubling history of eugenics reflects this thinking. Ending the life of a suffering person was framed in humanitarian and eugenic terms: the individual's relief from pain and suffering was coupled with the ideology of improving the race. These beliefs, along with claims about economic pragmatism and health management, are ideologies that authorize what Garland-Thomson calls the "cure-or-kill principle," whereby some bodies are eligible for rehabilitation and others classified as expendable. Persistent suffering becomes a sign of the inability to cope, compete, or control one's life. "The incurable body," she writes, "becomes an affront to the power of modern medical science and technology . . . a body that defies the sacred cultural ideologies of progress, self-determination, improvement, reform, and perfectibility—in other words, the very essence of what we take to be American."[13]

Throughout much of the twentieth century in America, under the logic of eugenics, "unfit bodies" were sequestered in hospitals, prisons, and asylums in order to maintain what Garland-Thomas refers to as "the fantasy of a normal, uniform, standardized, docile, and hygienic body."[14] However, the bodies of injured military veterans, *when they have been displayed in the service of demonstrating the efforts of physicians and scientists seeking novel ways of treating the ravages of war*, are an exception to this sequestering logic. While many languish in bureaucratically troubled veterans hospitals, out of the public's view, those whose bodies could dramatize the miracles of prosthetic technologies have been made hypervisible. What is remarkable is that bodies of war-injured U.S. veterans have been, since the emergence of photography, crucial in narratives of medical and, more recently, technoscientific salvation by which war is rationalized as valuable for human advancement. And this politics of visibility persists. It enacts war-generated biomedical technosalvationism in which the veteran's body-in-rehabilitation is a central visual trope.

Susan M. Schweik, in her historical analysis of laws that made it illegal for disabled people to appear in public, observes that disabled veterans of the U.S. Civil War were slightly more tolerated than other men who appealed for alms on city streets. But they were also doubted as malingerers who faked their disabilities or harmed themselves in order to avoid military service.[15] Following the Great War, "ugly laws" were invoked in the name of care for disabled veterans, keeping them from appearing in public so they wouldn't be confused with unworthy beggars. But the purpose of the ugly laws was also to prevent a kind of visual contamination or "influence" that would come from seeing abnormal bodies and persons. Given this history, what do we make of the now common display of veterans' war-wounded bodies in medical and popular journalism in our age of high-tech body enhancement, robotics, cyberprostheses, and regenerative medicine? It is no longer technically illegal for disabled people to be seen in public. In fact many of the images of wounded veterans from recent wars in Afghanistan and Iraq were valorized and circulated widely. These images were tethered to stories about biomedical advancements told in the grain of hegemonic framings of masculinity, valor, heterosexuality, and national sacrifice. They were exploited for garnering public support for "new and better" devices to overcome disfigurement and to affirm American technological know-how and patriotic belonging.

THE EMERGENT INDUSTRY OF BIONIC PROSTHETICS

Prosthetics research expanded substantially in the wake of the U.S. invasions of Afghanistan and Iraq, when the Department of Defense and the Veterans Administration became the largest funding sources.[16] Much of the research concerns bionics and robotics. Whereas bionics applies knowledge of biological systems to the design of technology, robotics combines methods from mechanical engineering, electrical engineering, and computer science to design machines capable of processing information and to perform tasks in response to sensory stimulation. Relying on biomimicry, the medical bionics industry makes artificial organs and builds limbs programmed with robotic locomotion that imitate natural systems of movement such as jumping, climbing, running, touching, handling, and grasping. By 2012 the global market value of the medical bionics industry was $12.67 billion, with the top five companies headquartered in North America.[17]

Prosthetics science valorizes the able body in historically shifting ways. Erin O'Connor argues that prosthetics science in Victorian culture was structured around metaphors of work, labor, strength, and productivity in a narrative framework of industrial capitalism. The clientele for artificial limbs were mainly men who had experienced industrial accidents and whose manhood was seen as compromised due to the injury. Therefore prosthetics science was geared toward restoring masculinity by putting the injured man's stump back to work and making him a productive laborer again, the ultimate sign of progress. As O'Connor writes, the prosthetic man became "a symbol of all that was possible in the modern world of manufacture, a walking advertisement for the personal and social benefits to be had from a full-scale embrace of machine culture."[18] Twenty-first-century prosthetics science extends this optimism within a narrative framework of post-Fordist capitalism in which the ideal worker is likened to an athlete who plays for the team and incorporates flexibility, physical fitness, and risk-taking in career choices.[19] These persons work on themselves to improve their value and productivity. Postmodern prosthetics science maintains an emphasis on individual achievement and overcoming bodily limitations while also incorporating chimerical aspects drawn from science fiction. Novel and lightweight materials, efficient power sources, and computerized neural-machine interfaces are assembled into bionic devices and attached to bodies with tissue regenerated by stem cells. Rather than being restored to its original condition, the body is imagined as a superior transmogrification.

Serlin, in his study of how physical rehabilitation became an allegory of national rehabilitation, argues that in the years following World War II medical procedures served as tools of consensus-building and promoted the idea that medicine was a leading method for domestic engineering. Prostheses from the period embodied cultural values concerning masculinity, productivity, and modernity.[20] The story goes back to the period after World War I, when rehabilitative medicine was enlisted to handle the ravages of combat and industrial accidents. This branch of medicine defined physical and sexual nonnormativity as no longer a personal badge of shame but instead a public health problem that could be studied and overcome. The rehabilitative prescription, applied to many afflicted persons, was to strive to become whole, to become beautiful, or to become the right kind of person and achieve the right kind of character. World War II further boosted the status of rehabilitative medicine since many veterans returned from war with shattered bodies, missing limbs, and psychological distress. Medical miracles touted in popular magazines during the relatively prosperous 1950s transformed procedures previously associated with emergency medicine or with elite society into consumer products for middle-class people interested in transforming their bodies and identities. Advertisements and magazine articles emphasized the benefits of military research that could "rebuild" humans, from new organ and blood banking procedures to replacement bladders, kidneys, and hearts, respirators, dialysis machines, and anti-aging therapies.

Serlin situates the development of prostheses for veteran amputees returning from World War II in the context of cultural anxieties about white masculinity, coinciding with publicized hand-wringing about what counted as proper behavior in the wake of the Kinsey studies on male sexuality.[21] Serlin argues that the design and development of prostheses during this period expressed the era's need to reengineer the physical body to accommodate the social mandates of the time. Focusing on the stainless steel split hook device designed by Henry Dreyfuss for the Veterans Administration, Serlin argues that the hand's functionalist quality and use of modern materials "represented the perfect armature with which veterans could challenge the emasculation often associated with their amputation." A new kind of subjectivity emerged in this process, in which some Americans who were able to change how they looked used new medical procedures and devices to become part of a national narrative in which "rehabilitating one's physical body made one more tangibly and visibly American than ever before."[22]

Likewise in the first decades of the twenty-first century, bionic engineering incorporated many of the dominant values of the larger context from which it emerged. New prostheses were designed to use computational algorithms to anticipate the users' needs, much the way Apple's voice-recognition technology Siri was designed to assist its human companions. Neurological circuits were engineered to link mechanical movement of artificial limbs to the cognitive and subconscious intentions of the user. Machine-assisted high-performance athletics and rehabilitative choreography reflected the corporate culture ideals of competition, teamwork, resilience, and entrepreneurial self-making. Models and simulations of intimacy refracted human-machine relationships through bionic prototypes of "feeling" robots that demonstrated technological wonder. Technophilic bromances formed between designers and engineers, overwhelmingly white men, who depended on injured bodies to form these bonds. Terrorist attacks could be surmounted by the loving care shared between an engineer and a victim of the Boston Marathon bombing whose love of dance helped to make her a beautiful survivor, an episode in this recent history to which I will return later in this chapter.

A new form of subjectivity emerged, expressed in a kind of distributive agency that pertains to the capacity of assemblages (bodies or selves) to affect and be effected by other kinds of bodies, including machines. This subjectivity dispenses with the monadic notion of one's "own" body or of the body as belonging to the self. Following Lisa Cartwright and Brian Goldfarb, I suggest that neural prosthetic use creates intrasubjective effects because, though users may refer to prostheses as "my legs" or "my arms," the assemblage is often described as a complex environment through which messages are conducted.[23] The brain-machine interface of neural prosthetics—limbs and parts controlled by messages sent from the brain through a microprocessor in the prosthetic—are enactments of what Jane Bennett calls vibrant matter that anachronize the notion of the possessing and "in control" individual.[24] The robobionic body assemblage can be thought of as an ecological or biotechnological system rather than a singular organic body rigged with a passive extension. This material-conceptual shift entails substantial ramifications for subjectivity and for how bionic subjects imagine and experience life, movement, frustrations, intimacy, and defeat. In some cases users complain that the bionic device is burdening rather than helping them. They are dissenters from the futuristic narrative of a seamless machine-body interface. Despite their makers' hopes, the technology is not incorporated by the user in these cases.

Though neural bionic technology promises to transmogrify even bodies that are not disabled, it continues to rest on a longer standing distinction between the normal and the exceptional body. However, rather than being banished, as in earlier eugenics logics, disability in bionics discourse becomes the grounds on which a kind of miraculous rebirth is imagined, provided the disabled is willing to participate in the drama of enhancement. Cassandra S. Crawford observes a hegemonic privileging of the able body in what she refers to as the discourse on prosthetized rebirth, a discourse that assumes the amputee body is a deficient body "amenable to liberatory enhancement and existential transcendence because it is 'in need of' technologic quickening." Its antithesis is the "normal" or "natural" body. Both bodies—"the deficient" and "the normal"—are moral, conceptual, technological, and practical co-constituted accomplishments in this discourse, not simply a priori or independent givens. Normality is always already being constructed. Within this discourse physical deficiency is "acquired" and then surmounted in an *achieved prosthetization*. While presenting itself in liberatory terms, prosthetized rebirth "asserts and affirms the distinction between the normal and the hybridized," securing exclusive biomedical authority in the researchers who "assume the role of the legitimate arbitrators of normality."[25] The dynamics of prosthetized rebirth are evident in military-funded projects aimed at integrating bionics, robotics, and artificial intelligence to produce a new generation of devices. Their development relies on the expertise of scientists but also, in large measure, on the wounded bodies of those returning veterans who demonstrated the will to be improved. Rather than being or becoming "normal" again, these are bodies whose profound injuries are the necessary condition for imagining (and valorizing) an elite of superpowered humans, resonant with cybernetically enhanced characters in the DC and Marvel comics Hollywood blockbuster movie franchises that gained immense popularity during the early twenty-first century. The X-Men, Batman, Superman, the Incredible Hulk, Iron Man, Captain America, Spider-Man, Ant-Man, the Fantastic Four, and Teenage Mutant Ninja Turtles take the concept of the Six Million Dollar Man and the Bionic Woman of the 1970s to new heights of enhancement.

While new bionic prosthetics science imagines bodies as assemblages mediated by neural phenomena that can be assisted by microprocessors, the bioengineers I focus on in this chapter each specialize in a particular part of the body and thereby establish expertise about the aesthetic form and practical function of that part. The artist-engineer David Hanson focuses on facial bionics. The biomechanical engineer Hugh Herr concentrates on lower limbs, and the neurological physician Geoff Ling on hands and arms. Compensating for losses in each of these body parts poses specific technological challenges for these inventors and the engineers with whom they collaborate.

MAKING FACES

Severely injured bodies returning home from Afghanistan and Iraq offered new opportunities for complex engineering projects through funding from various branches of the U.S. military. Among the most complicated parts of the body to rehabilitate is the human face. This is where Hanson's work comes into play. Hanson is among the leading bioengineers and materials scientists who received grants from the military to conduct research on making synthetic skin, building prosthetic ears and eyes, and engineering robotic facial expressions. Around the time he began his research, the state of the art was summarized by one science journalist as no better than what veterans of World War I were offered: reconstructive surgery, and if that proved inadequate or unviable, the patient was fitted with a mask whose function was limited to hiding the damage. Typically these earlier facial prostheses substituted for a single part, such as a nose, or a portion of the face that was damaged. A substitute nose, while it may not restore breathing or the sense of smell, could be a way to keep eyeglasses in place. But wearing a mask can also cause breath moisture to accumulate under it, which can steam up glasses and cause adhesive materials to slip. In recent years surgeons have approached these limitations with a goal of

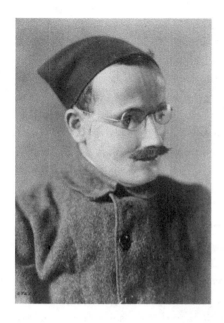

FIG 3.1 / Soldier with a mutilated face protected by a mask made by Anna Coleman Ladd, 1918. Courtesy of Library of Congress.

using advancements in organ transplant procedures to overcome them.[26] However, facial reconstruction remains challenging because of the complex organs and tissues that are necessary for seeing, hearing, breathing, eating, speaking, and making expressions. The face has intricate muscle systems that control the sinus and digestive tracts, breathing passageways, and ocular focus. Advancements in emergency medicine save people who would have died of severe facial injuries in the past. This accounts, in part, for why the military has invested heavily in this area of reconstructive medicine.

Dr. Maria Siemionow, an expert in plastic and microsurgery at the Cleveland Clinic, received military funding in 2008 to experiment with transplanting faces and limbs of laboratory rats and study the effects of immune rejection drugs. She investigated how to fuse donor and recipient cells to make "chimeric" cells that could act as immunomodulators so that recipients would not reject donated tissue. In 2008 a team she led performed the first "almost-full facial transplant" in the United States, three years after the first successful procedure had been done in France. The patients in both procedures were women, one who had been shot by her husband and the other who had overdosed on sleeping pills and was mauled by her dog while unconscious. The patients underwent multiple surgeries, were treated with drugs to suppress immune reactions, and had extensive physical therapy.[27] The hope was that the same procedure could be used to treat severely wounded veterans.

Two years earlier Hanson had received funding from DARPA to develop facial prostheses for U.S. soldiers returning from war with severe injuries. Rather than focusing on facial transplantation from a donor human to a patient, he was experimenting with simulating facial expressions by working with robot busts he designed. His work was not originally geared toward biomedical applications. When DARPA money became available, however, he reoriented his robotics research toward the goal of designing robotic masks to fit patients. During the 2006 PBS *NewsHour* segment, he explained that getting robots to make realistic facial expressions was a challenge. Another challenge presented itself when he began dealing with injured patients. "In order to restore the cosmetic appearance of an injured soldier's face, you need to fit the robotics to the face, while containing all of the power systems, motors and sensors within the appliance and have the appliance easy enough to maintain, be biocompatible, and able to mimic the soldier's remaining facial expressions so that the soldier can be able to control his or her face by thinking." Before all of this happens, though, he clarified that the patient's face would have to be surgically prepared to "accept the prosthesis." Using regenerative medicine techniques, laboratory workers would have to cultivate tissue compatible with the specific patient. The procedure would also involve a "smart bandage," consisting of sensors and a microfluid and pore system for oxygen circulation, in order to assist the healing of the "wounded environment." In other words, it would be a complicated process and a long time before the patient would actually receive an effective and custom-made prosthesis.

Hanson's work up to that point had little to do with medicine. He graduated in 1996 from the Rhode Island School of Design, where he studied sculpture and performance art. In a 1994 art school performance of *Sausage-Manhood* he played a macho character wearing BVD underwear "from which a 40-foot sausage protruded" and ran down College Street in Providence. During the performance the artist's sausage-manhood, according to Hanson, "starts to disintegrate as he runs and he seeks, in vain, to put it back together." He devolves into a "whining infantile state" and "keens for his loss of his Manhood, in a dance reflecting the plight of the ephemeral male ego and absurd trap of biological gender." Hanson described the project as "McCarthyesque," referring to his mentor, the iconoclastic performance artist Paul McCarthy.[28] In 2003 he went to UCLA to work with

McCarthy and was hired as an imagineer at Disney to create life-like figures for its theme parks. While pursuing a PhD in interactive arts at the
University of Texas at Dallas, he established Hanson Robotics, Inc. The
company's robots were designed for entertainment, teaching, and com-
panionship. Hanson concentrated on building faces and in a few years had
produced busts of a few people he admired: Einstein, Philip K. Dick, and
Alice-Eva, a robot based on his girlfriend at the time. By 2009 his company
had developed sixteen different "character robots," programmed with the
capacity to experience and express empathy. The robot heads were priced
at around $150,000 apiece.

In 2013 Hanson was commissioned by the billionaire Russian media
mogul Dmitry Itskov to design a robotic head. As the story goes, Itskov, at
the age of twenty-five, had a midlife crisis when he realized that he could
keep making lots of money and then just age and die, or he could try to
do something to remedy the way humans are "killing the planet." Instead
of charities to feed, clothe, and heal the poor, he thought charities could
be devoted to the goal of making affordable and long-lasting bodies. In
2013, at the age of thirty-two, he launched the Avatar Project. Also known
as the 2045 Initiative, the project's purpose is to upload human brains to
avatars, transferring consciousness from one body to another, using robotics to achieve immortality. Itskov said his goal was "to liberat[e] people
from death, from suffering, from the limits of biology." According to *Forbes*
magazine, the Dalai Lama endorsed the effort. The project envisioned four
processes to elude death: Avatar A was proposed as a robot that could be
controlled by a person's brain. Avatar B would be achieved once a brain
could be transplanted into a synthetic body. Avatar C would emerge after
the contents of a person's brain could be uploaded into a synthetic one.
Finally, Avatar D would be built as a hologram that replaced the body com-
pletely. According to Itskov's dream, future human bodies will not depend
on food or need shelter since they will be holograms. Health care, if you
want to call it that, will be geared toward repairing the new artificial body,
not the biological system.[29]

Martine Rothblatt, CEO of United Therapeutics, a biotechnology firm
that makes cardiovascular products, shares Itskov's aspirations. Rothblatt
is a transgender woman who worked first in the field of communication
and satellite law as CEO of Sirius XM Satellite Radio before turning to the
life sciences and the human genome project. In 2004 she wrote a popular
book on "xenotransplantation" and started the Terasem movement,

described in publicity materials as "a transhumanist school of thought focused on promoting joy, diversity, and the prospect of technological immortality via mind uploading and geoethical nanotechnology." In plainer terms, the school seeks to preserve individuals' consciousnesses in order to upload them into new bodies. Terasem is supported by a charitable foundation that holds meetings, makes public presentations, and publishes works explaining the framework of the movement. Rothblatt also authored *Mindfiles, Mindware and Mindclones*, a blog in which she writes about "the coming age of our own cyberconsciousness and techno-immortality."[30] Hanson approached Rothblatt in 2007. She subsequently commissioned him to build BINA48, a humanoid robot fashioned from Rothblatt's wife.[31] Millionaire benefactors' dreams of immortality helped to support Hanson's research on bionics and robotics. But the DARPA contract did more than provide him with funds; it offered a ground upon which to argue for bionic robotics in the rhetoric of care, compassion, and the repayment of the public's debt to those who had sacrificed their lives for the nation.

Hanson's team for the 2006 DARPA contract to rebuild faces consisted of artificial intelligence experts, hardware and software engineers, roboticists, and cognitive scientists whose mission was "to realize the dream of friendly machines who truly live and love, and co-invent the future of life."[32] Using "Identity Emulation," the team re-created real people, living or dead, in "robotic embodiments" that were portable. The process began with simulating humanlike facial features using Hanson's patented material, Frubber (face rubber), a spongy, porous, elastic polymer that mimics the movement of human musculature and skin through electroactive polymer actuators embedded in the robot's skin. The robot was equipped with microprocessors and artificial intelligence programming that enabled it to recognize faces and speech in order to carry on simple conversations. Its eyes contained micro-cameras to gather visual information for responding appropriately. It was able to emulate over sixty facial and neck muscle movements to form "approximately appropriate" facial expressions in response to specific stimuli. It smiled back when greeted by the researcher with a happy voice and smile. It looked sad when the researcher delivered unhappy news. During the many demonstrations that Hanson presented at TED Talks, tech conferences, and media interviews, the robot heads sat on pedestals or tables; the backs of the heads were exposed to show the circuitry and wires that powered them as Hanson interacted with them.

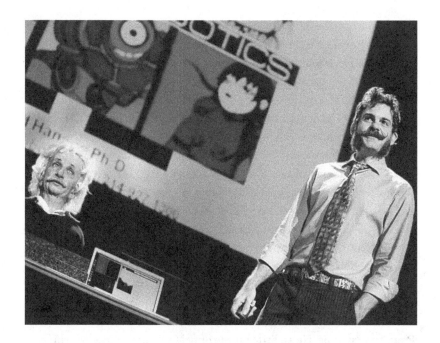

Critics accused Hanson of dehu-   FIG 3.2 / David Hanson with one of his
manizing life. He, however, described   genius machines.
his "genius machines" as enhancing
life. The first page of his online CV states, "In this age where most robots
are faceless and many are made for heartless military uses, I propose that
raising intelligent machines as endearing characters will prove key to making machines understanding and caring. Nurturing them among people
as works of art—living protagonists who befriend us and join the human
family—may push Artificial Intelligence to gain capabilities of compassion,
ethics, and general intelligence in ways familiar and comfortable to us. Such
machines may grow trustworthy and earn our love and respect." He insists
that his genius machines are no different from characters created by ani-
mators in films or novelists in fiction; they must have moral sensibilities,
"social intelligence," and above all, they must be believable. Humans, he asserts, are hardwired for social exchange. "There's a natural market pressure
for machines that have empathy, who like us, and even love us," he remarked
at an event called the Singularity Summit, a gathering of mainly young men
employed in the tech sector. He cited the success of this approach in *The
Sims* and *Second Life*, two massive online interactive digital games that are
populated by the emotionally complex avatars players create.

Hanson's vision of machine-enhanced life operates within an ontology of liberal humanism. This is typical of many researchers working on artificial intelligence and affective robotics. They occupy an echo chamber of repeated assumptions that ignore the realities of privilege and oppression supported by institutionalized power. Hanson does not distinguish between types of humans when he discusses what it is that he is attempting to mimic or simulate. The human remains an abstract entity that may be modified into "characters," but differences in social status that are structured by hierarchies of race, class, and gender are elided in his positing of the loveable and loving genius machines he makes. The imagineer does not take into account historical specificities that have enhanced the life chances of some human groups and vastly diminished those of others. He does not consider how experiences of racism and misogyny and class elitism shape how compassion and empathy are defined and have been used as tools of oppression. Hanson himself is an affable and even charming character in his TED Talks and interviews. His interactions with his genius machines are playful and sensitive, far from the evil and controlling Dr. Frankenstein type. He's a little bit Burning Man gonzo and a little bit sensitive New Age guy, with a leavening of postmodern steampunk mixed in. That he cares to do research that may help wounded veterans comes off as charitable and kind. It doesn't hurt that the biggest pot of money for this kind of research was held by the military itself.

LOWER-LIMB TECHNOLOGY: PERSONAL BIONICS AND INTIMATE EXTENSIONS

As wounded servicemen and -women returned home with severely damaged or amputated limbs, prosthetic engineers supported by funds from the Department of Defense continued to frame their research as an ethical response to the sacrifices made by these patients.[33] Innovators hoped not only to restore the body but also to transcend its normal limits. Otto Bock, a German company, received funding to advance its work in designing microprocessor knees. By 2009 it had developed X2, an artificial knee that allows its users to walk backward, ride a bike, and climb stairs. The knee is capable of determining its location in space and calculating how fast the user is moving. In 2009 the U.S. Army Medical Department began providing the device to amputees. In 2011 the company released a prototype of the more durable X3 knee that allows users to move in seawater and sand. The purchase price of an X3 is estimated at between $60,000 and $80,000 per unit, with the total cost to exceed $100,000 if a prosthetic foot is added.[34] Weighing a little less than three pounds, the X3 was designed to allow amputees to return to active duty. But the potential market is bigger. As one science journalist remarked, "All of these advances will also help millions of amputees who have never seen combat."[35] The suffering and sacrifices of veterans form the basis of an attachment to war, mediated through scientific research and prosthetics design that is accelerated as a consequence of war. Veteran amputees, returning from war, were central figures in narratives through which the public learned about the wonders of these new "smart limbs." The few who returned to active duty personified the miraculous nature of the technology and served to justify the military's large investment in this research area.

In 2004 the Department of Veterans Affairs gave Hugh Herr $7.2 million to create "biohybrid" limbs. Herr's company, iWalk, Inc., produced the PowerFoot One, an ankle-foot prosthesis that senses changing terrain and propels its user to push off the ground without expending as much energy as passive prostheses require.[36] The "veteran's ankle," as it is called, is equipped with five microprocessors, an electronic motor, and a measuring device that tracks its location in space and adjusts for walking up stairs or down inclines. Using sensors that were originally developed for guided missiles, the foot senses the ankle's location in space and adjusts the foot in order to walk forward, climb stairs and hills, or go down ramps. Next Herr licensed and commercially launched Rheo Knee, an artificial knee equipped with a microprocessor that senses the joint's position and the weight being applied to it and is able to adjust accordingly.

Herr had not worked with military patients prior to the wars in Afghanistan and Iraq, though he had been working on biomedical devices before the VA funded him. He founded the Biomechatronics Group at the Massachusetts Institute of Technology's Media Lab for interdisciplinary science projects that combine biology, mechanics, electronics, neuroscience, and robotics. In 2007 he trademarked the term *personal bionics* to denote "intimate extensions" of the body. What distinguishes personal bionics from passive prostheses is the incorporation of microprocessors programmed with the principles of muscle mechanics, neural control, and human biomechanics to assist in rehabilitation and to augment human physical capabilities "beyond what nature intended."[37] In 2013 Herr rebranded iWalk, Inc. as BiOM. As of June 2014 the BiOM board of directors included Herr and five other men who are associated with the company's main investors (WFD Ventures, General Catalyst Partners, Sigma Partners, and Gilde Healthcare Partners). The company had four executive officers, three men and one woman, with backgrounds in business management in the high-tech sector, engineering, kinesiology, and prosthetics sales and marketing. The VPs of sales and business development and marketing came from Össur Americas, a company founded in 1971 and headquartered in Iceland that specializes in bionic technology. It is named after Össur Kristinsson, an Icelandic prosthetist who developed a silicone interface for prosthetic sockets and the Symbionic Leg, "the world's first complete bionic leg incorporating Bionic Technology."[38] The Össur corporation developed many knee replacement devices and other products to reduce the pain and facilitate movement of patients suffering from osteoarthritis.

With military funding and seed money from private investment firms, Herr's BiOM company began manufacturing and selling the BiOM T2 Ankle System, a bionic propulsion device that replaces the lost muscle and tendon structure of the amputee's foot and propels the body by providing more energy than hydraulic or spring devices. Costing $50,000 apiece, the BiOM T2 mimics the human ankle, allowing transfemoral amputees to walk with what Herr's team calls a natural gait.[39] The team developed this technology in collaboration with colleagues at the VA Center for Excellence for Rebuilding, Regenerating and Restoring Function after Limb Loss in Providence, Rhode Island, the Spaulding Rehabilitation Hospital in Boston, and the Center for the Intrepid at Brooke Army Medical Center in San Antonio.

In 2007 the Center for the Intrepid opened a multidisciplinary occupational and physical rehabilitation facility to serve casualties coming back from Iraq and Afghanistan who had sustained amputations, burns, or functional limb loss. Its stated mission was to restore wounded service members with the possibility of returning those who are eligible to active duty. It accommodated research in orthopedics, prosthetics, and rehabilitation, provided inpatient and outpatient services, and had specialized labs for studying motion and gait deviations. In addition it had prosthetic fabrication and fitting specialists, virtual reality facilities for use in rehabilitation exercises, and firearms simulator training to reacquaint patients with weapons systems during their rehabilitation. The Center was funded with the help of donations from over 600,000 individual donors. As of 2012 the CFI served about six hundred patients a year.[40]

The VA and DoD helped Herr recruit research subjects who were war-wounded U.S. service members and veterans. In 2014 he acknowledged their dedication and contributions for the greater good, stating, "The U.S. warfighters' commitment to personal bionics has helped provide a more natural gait and normalized function to so many civilian individuals with lower-extremity amputation."[41] Herr's words echo the biomedical salvation narrative in his reference to the sacrifices military patients made for the nation, first in war and then, as research subjects, in performing the duty of rehabilitation. In both modalities, the research subjects simultaneously served the nation and biomedical advancement by participating in rehabilitative therapies that would benefit civilians too.

Herr was keen to develop neuroprostheses—devices that would integrate the mind, body, and machines by emulating sensory feedback loops found in human physiology. He teamed up with researchers at Brown University and the Providence Veterans Administration Center. Team member John Donoghue concentrated on the brain-machine interface and developed a system called BrainGate to decode brain waves in order to translate them into computer commands. Donoghue explained that the BMI (brain-machine interface) works by having an output function that goes from the brain to the body part via a neural interface that first detects the neurally coded intent. Then it decodes this into a movement command that drives a physical device (such as a computer) or a body part (such as a paralyzed limb) so that the intent becomes an action. The BMI's input from the paralyzed limb to the brain occurs through a stimulus that is detected by a physical device, coded into a signal, and then delivered via the interface to the user to elicit a proper percept (i.e., touch or vision). The user determines the use of the inputs and outputs through a voluntary interplay between the percept and desired action.[42] A microsensor is implanted in a part of the brain that controls movement.

Cartwright and Goldfarb describe neural prostheses as "neither iconic and substantive nor supplemental and facilitative." Instead, they argue, these prostheses afford a new kind of agency that arises from the brain and nervous system controlling the prosthetic device. The device "is not a medium but materially reconfigures the intersubjective unit body and technology as an *intrasubjective* entity." In this way agency is "radically and synthetically distributed and *interconstitutive* within the unitary body," and consciousness is key to this "neural configuration."[43] However, the condition of the user's consciousness matters to the efficacy of use. In severely brain-damaged amputees, neural prostheses have to be designed to take these conditions into account. Likewise they need to be custom-fit to the body to facilitate movement. The result is a complex intrasubjective reorientation of thoughts to actions through the patient's dependence upon a computer to read his or her brain's intentions. Adapting to the assemblage is challenging for many patients. In an early BMI test conducted by Herr, one quadriplegic patient was able to switch on lights by using his brain to generate thoughts that the computer translated. But the apparatus was awkward, consisting of many wires that attach to the patient's head. This spurred the team to begin work on a wireless implant system that would allow the patient to direct hand and leg movements with signals sent from the brain. Herr's persistent hope that the computer could learn from the brain how it is supposed to direct the prosthetic device means that his prototypes may not be useful for patients with brain damage or severe mental distress.

Herr collaborated with researchers at Northwestern University and the Rehabilitation Institute of Chicago on ways to connect prostheses to the central nervous system so that a user would be able to operate the device just by thinking, using BIONS (bionic neurons). Team member Todd Kuiken developed a technique called targeted muscle reinnervation, which consists of surgically connecting "orphaned" nerves to the amputee's remaining muscles. Once these nerves are connected, the muscles contract in response to signals from the brain that go out to the absent limbs. The muscle contractions are sensed by electrodes attached to the skin near the muscles, which in turn send a signal to the microprocessor of the Power-Foot to flex the artificial foot.

The VA also funded Herr and Richard Weir for a collaborative project to develop the Implantable Myoelectric Sensor (IMES), a wireless device developed by Weir and two other engineers that uses a software program to connect nerves and muscles with the goal of allowing amputees to control prostheses.[44] For lower-limb amputees, a small incision is made in what remains of the amputee's leg and two microchips are implanted in the residual muscle that leads to the front and back of the calf. Fibrous tissue holds the implants in place. When the muscles contract, the sensor transmits a signal to the PowerFoot through the wireless system, enabling the prosthesis to move the ankle. The IMES uses signal-processing algorithms to translate the signals into the intended movements of the user, allowing users to control the prosthetic with their own muscles.

FROM A BLIZZARD COMES A WIZARD

Herr is a particularly compelling spokesperson for bionic science. In his early twenties he suffered frostbite after getting lost in a blizzard while climbing in the White Mountains of New Hampshire with a friend. The frostbite caused the amputation of both his legs below the knee. A common narrative refrain in media interviews is that the experience spurred this avid rock climber to figure out better ways to design prostheses than the clunky plaster-of-paris limbs and cane he was given after his amputation.[45] Necessity was the mother of invention. Its two main inventions were a family of ever-improving prostheses and a new identity for the young survivor of frostbite. He was prosthetically born again.

By his own account, before the accident Herr was a high school student with a dismal grade point average, more interested in hiking and rock climbing than he was in school. He told one reporter that while attending vocational night school in rural Pennsylvania he "didn't know what 10 percent of 100 was."[46] The accident changed all this. After his injury Herr started experimenting with making more functional devices than were available to him. He designed a pair of legs made from aluminum tubes with special feet that were good for rock climbing and much lighter in weight than the plaster legs. Three years after the accident Jeff Batzer, a friend who was also injured in the climbing accident, introduced him to Barry Gosthnian, a former air force mechanic in Vietnam who had become an orthotist and prosthetist. Gosthnian was in the process of developing a hydraulic cushion with shock-absorbing capability to place between the knee and a prosthetic leg. He got the idea from working with aircraft landing gear. Herr and Batzer worked with Gosthnian to develop an improved socket. Herr headed off to college to become a math and science major, and a few years later he shared his first patent with Gosthnian for a prototype of a cushion socket using inflatable bladders made out of compliant polyurethane. According to most accounts, his accident was a catalyst to defy the doctors' prediction that he would never run or climb again and to become a scientist who would go on to earn an MS in mechanical engineering at MIT and a PhD in biophysics from Harvard. Overcoming the odds, he is an exemplar of twenty-first-century resilient and enterprising ingenuity.

In 2007 he co-organized a symposium with the radio journalist and disability rights activist John Hockenberry titled H2.0: New Minds, New Bodies, New Identities at the MIT Media Lab. Hockenberry's car accident at the age of twenty left him paralyzed from the midchest down, a subject he wrote about in his acclaimed *Moving Violations: War Zones, Wheelchairs and Declarations of Independence*. The MIT symposium was announced in grandiose prose:

> The story of civilization is the story of humans and their tools. Use of tools has changed the human mind, altered the human body, and fundamentally reshaped human identity. Now at the dawn of the twenty-first century, a new category of tools and machines is poised to radically change humanity at a velocity well beyond the pace of Darwinian evolution. A science is emerging that combines a new understanding of how humans work to usher in a new generation of machines that mimic or aid human physical and mental capabilities. Some 150 million of us are over the age of 80, while 200 million of us suffer from severe cognitive, emotional, sensory, or physical disabilities. Giving all or even most of this population a quality of life beyond mere survival is both the scientific challenge of the epoch and the basis for a coming revolution over what it means to be human. To unleash this next stage in human development, our bodies will change, our minds will change, and our identities will change. The age of Human 2.0 is here.

Invited participants included the paralympic athlete and performance artist Aimee Mullins, the neuroscientist John Donoghue, and the famous neurologist and best-selling author Oliver Sacks. Much of the daylong conference focused on rethinking the distinction between "able bodied" and "disabled bodies" in light of new technologies that bring together neural processes and computing. Panelists discussed research in music and neural processing, social robotics, memory augmentation, and neuroprosthetics for treating depression and motor-neuron diseases.[47]

Herr's enthusiasm for generating new thinking about body enhancement was infectious. He became a rock star in the emergent field of biomechatronics, was featured on the cover of *Wired* magazine, and was invited to present his work at TED events. During a 2014 TED Talk he gave in Vancouver, he began by telling his audience that bionic devices were beginning to bridge the gap between disability and ability, between human limitation and human potential. With a large photograph of a rock climber projected behind him, Herr walked deliberately around the stage, establishing eye contact and saying, "Bionics has defined my physicality. [After my accident]

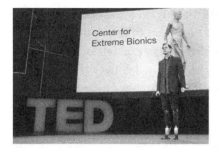

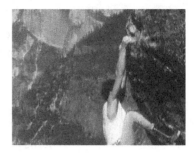

I didn't view my body as broken. I reasoned that a human being can never be broken. Technology is broken. Technology is inadequate. This

FIG 3.3 / Hugh Herr giving a TED Talk.

FIG 3.4 / Hugh Herr climbing with his bionic legs.

simple but powerful idea was a call to arms to advance technology for the elimination of my own disability and ultimately the disability of others." In Herr's phenomenology, "the artificial part of my body is malleable, able to take on any form, any function, a blank slate through which to create structures that can extend beyond biological capability." He credited technology with allowing him to return to his favorite sport stronger and better than ever, through the use of spiked prosthetic feet and narrow-wedge prosthetic feet that enable him to climb vertical ice walls and steep rock fissures. "Technology had eliminated my disability and allowed me a new climbing prowess." But technology, he added, had a lot of room for improvement: "Sadly, because of deficiencies in technology, disabilities are rampant in the world."[48] Technological salvation is at the center of Herr's public presentations: disabilities exist because existing technology is deficient. Eliminate these deficiencies with properly functioning technology and disabilities disappear.

Herr's Vancouver TED Talk was part didactic lecture, part testimonial performance art, roughly in equal proportions. He used his own body and his bionic legs as a "case in point" to illustrate the MIT Media Lab's Center for Extreme Bionics' mission of advancing "fundamental science and technological capability that will allow the biomechatronic and regenerative repair of humans across a broad range of brain and body disabilities." He spent a good deal of the standard TED Talk eighteen-minute format explaining how his legs work, delineating the three "extreme interfaces" that pertain to his bionic limbs: the mechanical (how his limbs are attached to his biological body), the dynamic (how they move like flesh and bone), and the electrical (how they communicate with his nervous system). Projected above him was what he referred to as the "beautifully lyrical design work" of an MIT colleague depicting "spatially-varying exoskeletal impedances" rendered in color variation by a 3-D-printed model. Herr explained how bionic limbs are attached to biological bodies through synthetic skins that can stiffen or relax to provide optimum support and flexibility, like clothing. Tissue compliance is achieved, he continued, through mathematical modeling, MRI imaging of the geometries and locations of various tissues inside the body, and the use of robotic tools to measure tissue compliances at various anatomical points. Where the body is stiff, the synthetic skin should be soft; where the body is soft, the synthetic skin should be stiff to protect the joints against high impact. The result is that "we have produced bionic limbs that are *the* most comfortable limbs I've ever worn."

THE TED TALK PHENOMENON

Since so many of the cutting-edge ideas about bionics are transmitted via TED Talks, I want to take a moment here to discuss the genre and the organization with which it is associated before returning to the specifics of Herr's TED Talk. The TED organization began in 1984 as a conference focused on the convergence of "Technology, Entertainment, and Design." By the second decade of the twenty-first century it was referring to itself as "a global community." TED's founder is an American architect and designer, Richard Saul Wurman, who turned it over to the British technology publishing entrepreneur Chris Anderson in 2002. By his own account, Anderson had experienced a midlife crisis caused by the dot-com crash of the late 1990s as he lost $1 million of his net worth each day. The experience led him to seek more meaningful ways to think about the future than he had while working in the tech industry. In 2001 he established the Sapling Foundation and gradually acquired TED as a program of the foundation. In its promotional material TED's mission is to "spread ideas" through this "global clearinghouse of free knowledge from the world's most inspired thinkers—a community of curious souls to engage with ideas and each other." Anderson served as its "curator," a term that replaced the more conventional chief executive officer.

There is much talk of "passion," "curiosity," "creative disruption," and "gurus" in the TED organization's promotional materials and among its participants. The organization holds an annual large convention as well as specialized TEDx events around the United States and abroad. TEDMED Talks, for example, focus on health and medical technologies. TED Talks began appearing online in 2006, as video-sharing sites and social media started to proliferate. While designed to be accessible and entertaining, all the TEDx science and health talks are required to comply with guidelines stipulating that any information that is conveyed must be supported by peer-reviewed research. The organization describes itself as nonpartisan. It gives out an annual prize and supports a TED fellows program that "supports extraordinary new voices as they develop their careers in science, the arts, social justice and more."

TED has headquarters in New York City and Vancouver. The TED website lists members of "the TED Brain Trust," who provide advice on issues of importance to TED's future. Among the thirty-three listed on the site in May 2014 were Bill Gates, founder of Microsoft; Jeff Bezos, founder of Amazon; Larry Page and Sergey Brin, cofounders of Google; Ray Kurzweil, a "futurist" and director of engineering at Google; and the musician Peter Gabriel. Members of the Brain Trust were identified by a variety of conventional as well as eccentric designations: artist, social psychologist, university chancellor, philanthropist, design guru, philosopher, psychologist, inventor, physicist, CEO, architect, futurist, software visionary, IP innovator, polymath, musician, marketing guru, creativity expert, venture capitalist, evolutionary psychologist, connector extraordinaire, marine biologist, and anthropologist. The majority of the members were U.S. citizens. Eight of the thirty-three were women. Most of the academics were associated with elite universities (Stanford, MIT, Harvard). All but three were white people, including the eight women. The three were Ashraf Ghani, an Afghan national and chancellor of Kabul University; John Maeda, a Japanese American computer scientist and designer; and Juan Enriquez, a Mexican national who negotiated a cease-fire with the Zapatistas for the Mexican government. While claiming to be global, the organization is overwhelmingly dominated by white American elite-educated men who have made fortunes in the technology sector.

I think of TED as a kind of secular technosalvationist tent revival circuit of the arrived and the up-and-coming, with lip service paid to the empty-and-everything tropes of diversity and inclusion. I am sympathetic to Benjamin Bratton's scathing critique of TED Talks performed in his own TED Talk, where he argued that the group's acronym didn't really stand for Technology, Entertainment, and Design but for "Middlebrow Megachurch

Infotainment." Staying within the standard eighteen-minute format, Bratton accused TED of encouraging oversimplification of complex ideas, a tendency toward showmanship at the expense of substance, an inclination toward "placebo politics" and "placebo innovation" (i.e., excessive faith in technology to solve problems), and an affective habit of blending epiphany and personal testimony ("epiphimony") "through which the speaker shares a personal journey of insight and realization."[49] Nathan Jurgenson similarly objected to TED Talks' epistemic style for having a limited understanding of what counts as knowledge and how that knowledge is disseminated, arguing that it is out of touch and exclusionary and disavows its own corporatist allegiances.[50]

Now let's get back to what Herr was saying at that Vancouver convention about overcoming the limits of existing prosthetic technology in 2014.

BIONIC SALVATION: FROM AFGHANISTAN
TO THE BOSTON MARATHON

During his presentation, a video clip features a man running up a rocky pathway as Herr explains how the bionic limbs he is wearing were given to nearly a thousand patients, four hundred of them wounded U.S. soldiers. We learn that the man in the clip lost his legs in a bomb blast while serving in Afghanistan. Another clip shows a man with "normal physiology" on a treadmill wearing an exoskeletal structure that augments human walking by significantly reducing metabolic cost. Bionics such as these, Herr explains, will make us all stronger and faster and more efficient. "It's so profound in its augmentation," he continues, "that when a normal healthy person wears the device for more than 40 minutes and then takes it off, their own biological legs feel ridiculously heavy and awkward." As he picks up the pace from walking to running in place before the audience, Herr smiles and tells them he feels great. The crowd applauds with enthusiasm.

Herr's preferred vision of the future is one in which rigorous scientific calculation offers superior solutions to "artisan strategies" that have dominated prosthetic design but, in his view, have hindered rather than enhanced ability. The new "data-driven" products promise to deliver us all from a host of problems, whether obesity, attention-deficit disorder, schizophrenia, traumatic brain injury, multiple sclerosis, sleep disorders, Parkinson's disease, or depression. These words flash on a screen behind him during the TED talk, as he articulates the claim that "every person should have the right to live life without disability if they so choose. We, the people, need not accept our limitations but can transcend disability through technological innovation. And indeed through fundamental advances in bionics in this century, we will set the technological foundation for an enhanced human experience and we will end disability."

Scholars of disability studies and activists working for the rights and liberation of disabled people have criticized this kind of technological triumphalism on a number of grounds, chiefly arguing that many disabilities are not readily remedied or substantially mitigated by technology. In addition disability rights advocates point to the rhetoric of "eliminating" disabilities as reminiscent of eugenics, which championed the idea of exterminating those whose disabilities made their lives "not worth living." Another line of critique argues that technological triumphalism degrades the cultural identities and communities of people living with "differently abled" bodies. Deaf activists and advocates of Deaf culture, for example, have argued that cochlear implants pathologize deafness while eroding the unique expressive qualities of sign language.[51] Herr's position is somewhat nuanced compared with that of cochlear implant advocates because, unlike cochlear implants, his bionic devices do not require invasive and painful surgery, and restoring one's ability to walk is arguably not the same as culturally degrading Deaf culture and language. Furthermore, like many disabled rights advocates, Herr seeks to redefine the term *disability* by suggesting that it is human-made environments and flawed prosthetic devices that are themselves disabling. As this line of reasoning goes, if things were built and made differently, many people previously considered disabled would be able to function and even thrive. However, critics of this position argue that certain disabilities (and the bodily or material conditions in which they place people) are so profound that they cannot be "fixed" away by technology or changes in spatial design. From this perspective, Herr would be seen as advocating a variant of assimilationist politics in which disabilities can and should "disappear" through engineered interventions. Others argue that rather than assuming we can eradicate disabilities, we should move away from notions of the perfect (and enhanced) body. They might criticize Herr for advancing a framework that insists people should challenge themselves to improve their conditions and that assumes those who do not are foolishly resisting the promising future of technological salvationism.[52]

Herr's 2014 talk ends with a dramatic coda in which he tells the story of Adrianne Haslet-Davis, a young woman who "breathes and lives dance"

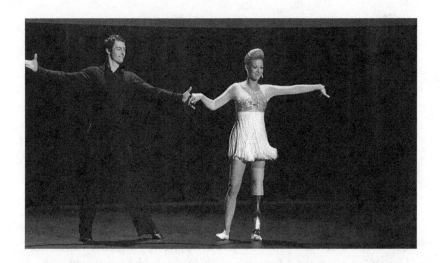

and for whom dance is "her expression, her art form." The two met at
the Harvard-related Spaulding Rehabilitation Center in Boston, where

FIG 3.5 / Adrianne Haslet-Davis and
partner during Hugh Herr's Vancouver
TED Talk.

Herr was seeing patients. Haslet-Davis was at Spaulding recovering from
losing her left leg. Her story entangles biomedicine with the Global War
on Terror as it shook the city of Boston. On April 15, 2013, she was near
the finish line at the Boston Marathon when a pair of homemade bombs
exploded, planted by a pair of brothers who had emigrated to the United
States with their parents from Kyrgyzstan in 2002 and 2004.[53] Learning of
Haslet-Davis's passion for ballroom dancing, Herr decided to assemble his
team to build her a bionic limb so she could dance again. The team studied the movement of dancers for six months, drawing on data about the
principles of dance and imbedding them into the new bionic limb. While a
video during Herr's TED Talk shows an animated skeleton and a real dancer
carrying out the same movements, Herr emphasizes the power of technology to stand up to terrorists and to advance humanity: "Bionics is not only
about making people stronger and faster. Our expression, our humanity
can be embedded into electromechanics. It was 3.5 seconds between the
bomb blast in the Boston terrorist attack and 3.5 seconds the criminals
and cowards took Adrianne off the dance floor. In 200 days, we put her
back. We will not be intimidated, brought down, diminished, conquered,
or stopped by acts of violence. [Applause.] Ladies and gentlemen, please
allow me to introduce Adrianne Haslet-Davis, her first performance since

the attack." She comes out from the wings with a dance partner, and they dance for about a minute with graceful but slightly tentative movements to Enrique Iglesias's "Ring My Bells." The audience erupts in applause; she wipes away a tear and gives Herr a kiss and a hug. The dancers, Herr, and two other members of the research team—arm in arm—together take a bow in this collective performance.

Haslet-Davis, as a cultural figure, shares something with the war-wounded soldier under the clinical observation of Herr's team: both embody survival, resilience, and dedication; both demonstrate the promising horizon of technological enhancement of the body; and both suture the enhanced body to the hegemonic narrative of national strength.

THE CHALLENGE OF UPPER-LIMB PROSTHETICS

Compared to legs, upper limbs are far more complex in their function and capability. To fulfill the minimum daily requirements of movement, a leg needs what orthotic and prosthetic engineers refer to as four "degrees of freedom." An upper-body limb requires twenty-two degrees.[54] Shoulders and wrists normally rotate. Wrists, shoulders, and elbows extend and flex. Fingers are able to pick up small objects and do a wide variety of fine motor activities—everything from writing, painting, typing, sewing, knitting, carving, and gardening to playing musical instruments. They are also more sensitive to temperature, touch, and pain than lower limbs or feet. Hands have about twenty muscles to control movement. Arms have about seventy thousand nerve fibers that connect to the spinal cord. Building a functionally replaceable upper limb is much more challenging than building a lower limb because of these complex operations.

For over a century and a half, dating from the mid-nineteenth century, prosthetic upper-body limbs resembled split hooks, attached by a shoulder harness to the torso and powered by the body of the wearer. The split hook patented by David Dorrance in 1912 came to be the standard-bearer for most of the twentieth century. It operated on a cable pulley system and allowed the user to open and close the "finger" and "thumb" of the hook, functioning like a pair of tweezers. Although many upper-limb amputees continue to favor it over a new generation of neural-interfacing artificial arms, engineers working with DARPA's Revolutionizing Prosthetics program frequently lamented that upper-limb prosthetic technology lagged considerably behind lower-limb devices.

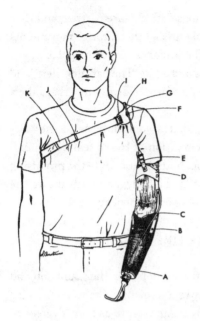

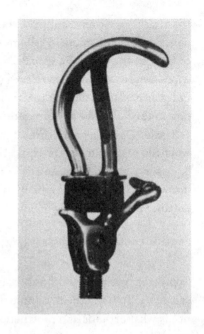

DARPA's interest in biological and medical sciences dates back to the mid-1990s, when the Pentagon learned that enemies could develop biological weapons with relative ease and expense. Its interest coincided with the rapid expansion of the biotechnology industry during the 1990s. DARPA's

FIG 3.6 / The Dorrance hook, 1912, designed by D. W. Dorrance, who lost his arm in an industrial accident in 1909. From Bender, *Prosthesis and Rehabilitation after Arm Amputation*.

FIG 3.7 / Close-up of the Dorrance hook, 1912. From Bender, *Prosthesis and Rehabilitation after Arm Amputation*.

investment in biological science was eventually consolidated in 2014 in its new Biological Technologies Office.[55] The Revolutionizing Prosthetics program became a unit of that office and was where DARPA's Bio-Revolution programs were administered. A DARPA communications officer explains, "All of DARPA's Bio-Revolution programs have one mission in mind: to use the life sciences to benefit the U.S. military and to save American lives."[56]

Described by its director as an arms race of a different sort, the Revolutionizing Prosthetics program addressed the challenges of building upper-limb prosthetics that function like arms and hands and resemble them visually more than the "hook on a stick" design. DARPA-funded bionic arms perform a wider range of activities by relying on microprocessors and neural signaling technologies and using the muscles of the chest to substitute for missing arm muscles.

The precursor to the Revolutionizing Prosthetics program was DARPA's Human Assisted Neural Hand Devices program, established in 2002, involving scientists from Duke University and the University of Pittsburgh whose research demonstrated that the brain's neural signals could be captured, decoded, and used to drive a peripheral device. The researchers worked with nonhuman primates to demonstrate the ability to operate prosthetic hands that can reach and grasp based upon signals extracted and decoded from the motor cortex.[57] Building on this earlier research, within six years the Revolutionizing Prosthetics program had developed two "anthropomorphic advanced modular prototype arm systems"—devices that incorporated sockets for increasing the range of motion of arms and hands, enabling dexterity, and offering more control options.[58] The prototypes were developed quickly in response to an uptick in injured troops returning from Iraq and Afghanistan.

In 2006 DARPA awarded $30.4 million to the Applied Physics Lab at Johns Hopkins University to develop another advanced arm system that would use the brain to control the neuroprosthetic limb. This second main product of the Revolutionizing Prosthetics program was announced in 2012. The goal of the research was to design a prosthetic limb connected directly to the peripheral and central nervous system so that users would be able to operate the arm and hand with signals from the brain. Working with tetraplegic volunteers, researchers sought to demonstrate the value of the device for patients suffering from upper-limb paralysis. In September 2011 they conducted a test in which one of the volunteers was able to control the biomechanical arm by using his brain signals recorded by electrocorticography. By the summer of 2014 DARPA had contracted more than $107 million to the Hopkins Lab to develop and improve the neuroprosthetic arm.

As the wars in Afghanistan and Iraq wore on and public support for them was flagging, military public affairs officers sent out press releases announcing medical innovations coming out of newly established research consortia. The message was familiar: war is terrible, but we are dedicating our best scientific talent to dealing with the wounds suffered by those who have risked their lives for the defense of the nation. Researchers were portrayed as heroes on the front lines of war at home. The discourse of debt, redemption, and salvation resonated in media coverage of biomedical prosthetic design. Salvaged bodies of injured veterans were central to a narrative of bodily enhancement that would take humans into a future beyond the limitations of our "natural" bodies. Enhancement was the new and improved normal. Telling the story to a receptive and indebted audience was part of the public relations strategy of the Pentagon, especially during a time when scandals about the bureaucratic neglect at Walter Reed and other military hospitals were making headline news. News stories about the alarming rates of untreated PTSD and suicide among returning troops contributed to the bad reputation of military medical facilities. Miraculous devices, public affairs officers hoped, would overshadow the unseemly news about veterans being poorly cared for or dying while waiting to get an appointment to see a doctor.

POPULARIZING A NEW ARMS RACE

In April 2009, 60 *Minutes* aired a story on the Pentagon's bionic arm. The segment begins with reporter Scott Pelley explaining:

> When Americans are wounded in Afghanistan and Iraq, no expense is spared to save their lives. But once they are home, if they have suffered an amputation or lose their arm, they usually end up wearing an artificial limb that hasn't changed much since World War Two. In all the wonders of modern medicine, building a robotic arm with a fully functioning hand has not been remotely possible but that is starting to change. You're about to see a remarkable leap in technology called the DEKA Arm. And, as we first reported this past spring, it is just one of the breakthroughs in a $100 million Pentagon program called Revolutionizing Prosthetics. To see how far they've come, take a look at how they started.[59]

The camera cuts to an upper-limb amputee in a suit and tie explaining how his "basic hook" works by rotating it and locking it. The man is Fred Downs, a veteran who stepped on a land mine in Vietnam in 1968 and lost his arm. By 2009 he was the head of prosthetics for the Veterans Administration.

We next meet Dr. Geoffrey Ling, an intensive-care physician who specializes in treating traumatic brain injury and who served two combat tours in Iraq and Afghanistan. Moved by caring for Afghan children, Ling joined DARPA because it "had the money and minimal bureaucracy." Things could get done fast. He describes DARPA's Revolutionizing Prosthetics program as a project of imperial benevolence. In a separate interview he tells a science journalist, "It's America again doing the best things that America can do, which is showing that . . . we are a superpower that really tries to take care of the world."[60] In another interview Ling notes, "At DARPA, we have a vision of a future where a soldier who has lost an extremity in battle will regain full use of that limb again. We will get to this future by making revolutionary, neurally controlled prosthetics. . . . We will do whatever is necessary to restore these people who have given up so much for the idea of freedom and in service to their country."[61] In a 2014 press release, he was quoted saying that he launched the Revolutionizing Prosthetics program to provide better care "to repay some of the debt that we owe to our Service members."[62] The biomedical salvation narrative, according to which American citizens owe a debt to wounded troops and war provides the conditions for advancing knowledge and making the world better, is captured in Ling's earnest claims.

The 60 Minutes camera crew follows the doctor through a rehabilitation clinic where physical therapists assist wounded veterans as Pelley narrates: "He's a physician with big dreams and little patience, especially when touring Walter Reed Army Medical Center and meeting the troops he's working for." During a seated interview Ling explains the complexity of the human hand, with its opposable thumb and four fingers that move independently of one another. Pelley interjects, "And if you lose your hand you lose part of being human."

"You're so right, Scott!" Ling responds. "Think about what makes us separate from any other animal species. We have an opposable thumb. That is a fact that makes us human," forgetting that nonhuman primates, raccoons, and koala bears also have opposable thumbs.

"Colonel Ling," Pelley intones in the voice-over narrative, "is determined to give that humanity back. His project is run out of DARPA, the same group that saw the creation of night vision [goggles], stealth aircraft, and GPS." In the 60 Minutes script DARPA is thanked for innovations that are now part of everyday life for many watching the show. And as DARPA turns its focus to bioengineering, this notoriously secretive and wildly extravagant funding source that is responsible for some of the most deadly weapons systems ever devised is able to appear benevolent and caring because of its association with medicine and healing.

"Give me a sense of the scale of this project," Pelley requests.

"It's a very large scale," Ling answers, "very much like the Manhattan Project in that scope. It's an over $100 million investment now and it involves well over 300 scientists."

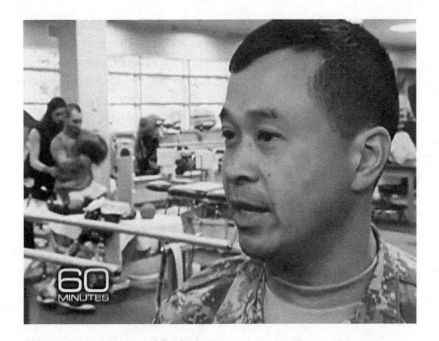

Pelley then introduces Dean Kamen, "a sort of rock star of inventors
who flies his own jet." We see Pelley with Kamen operating a remote-
control device in what looks like a
small airport. "It's the fastest non-military airplane that you can buy any-
where in the world," Kamen remarks, while remotely taxiing the jet out of
the hangar. Pelley tells us that Kamen invented dozens of medical devices
in addition to his most famous invention, the Segway scooter—"inventions that have made him a multimillionaire." We watch the two riding the
self-balancing Segways along a well-groomed park, somewhere near the
DEKA Research and Development Corporation in Manchester, New Hampshire, where Kamen is the chief executive officer.

FIG 3.8 / Geoffrey Ling being interviewed as a veteran is assisted in rehab
exercises by a trainer. From "The Pentagon's Bionic Arm," *60 Minutes*, 2009.

Kamen cofounded the company in 1982 at the age of thirty-one, and by
then had already developed and patented the Auto-syringe, the first portable infusion device for delivering drugs that once required around-the-
clock hospital care. He grew up on Long Island, the son of Jack Kamen, an
illustrator for MAD magazine, *Weird Science*, and other comics. A college
dropout, the younger Kamen nevertheless supported education through
his nonprofit organization, FIRST (For Inspiration and Recognition of

Science and Technology). Founded in 1989, FIRST aims to inspire teenagers to pursue careers in science. Kamen has given frequent TED Talks, including a 2007 talk titled "Luke, a New Prosthetic Arm for Soldiers." He named the device after Luke Skywalker, whose hand was sliced off by Darth Vader's laser saber in *The Empire Strikes Back*. After he loses his hand, Luke is on a medical spaceship and a robot checks the sensation of his new prosthetic hand. The miraculous scene inspired Kamen to memorialize it in the naming of his DEKA Arm System. DARPA gave Kamen $18.1 million to make the device.

"When the folks from the Defense Department came to this office and said 'here's what we need,' what did you tell them?" asks Pelley.

Kamen replies, "We want these kids to have something put back on them that will essentially allow one of these kids to pick up a razor or a grape off the table and know the difference without looking at it. That is an extraordinary goal."

Researchers in the study observed activities and gathered feedback from thirty-six military amputees. Out of this effort the Gen-3Arm System was tested and refined. In April 2012 DEKA submitted a 501(k) premarket notification to the Food and Drug Administration seeking approval to make the Arm System commercially available. USAMRMC added funding to complete the necessary tests and trials required by the FDA. The DARPA press release for the DEKA Arm System noted that the hand could allow service members to return to duty and could also be used by robots for unexploded ordnance removal, thus limiting the risks currently faced by soldiers assigned to such duties. From its inception in 2006, DARPA set a goal of gaining FDA approval for an advanced electromechanical prosthetic upper limb with "near-natural" control so that amputees could gain greater independence and have an improved quality of life. In a little less than eight years the FDA approved the DEKA Arm System for general use in May 2014.[63]

Kamen guides Pelley through the production site, explaining how his team of forty engineers spent a year working on the problem and came up with the DEKA Arm, equipped with gears, joints, and microprocessors that mimic "nature's design." The persistent problem was that the arm weighed too much (nine pounds), and this was likely to result in "prosthetic abandonment," a typical outcome for many upper-limb amputees who find it awkward, uncomfortable, painful, or too cumbersome to wear poorly designed prosthetic devices.[64] To address this problem Kamen's team interviewed patients at Walter Reed and similar facilities and realized they would have to design a way for the DEKA Arm to be lighter and to connect with the body more effectively. In response the team developed tiny balloons that assisted movement by inflating and deflating as the wearer uses the arm to do tasks such as grasping, reaching, holding, and releasing.

Fred Downs, the Vietnam War veteran and head of the VA prosthetics branch, demonstrates the DEKA Arm attached to his shoulder by a strap and belt. He says he's skeptical after years of seeing inventions come and go and experiencing firsthand the body's limited tolerance for gadgetry. He controls the DEKA Arm by flexing his shoulder and pressing buttons that are built into his shoes, using the toes to "type" out the commands. Pelley announces, "After practicing for ten hours, Downs showed us what he could do." We watch Downs pick up a soda bottle and start to drink from it. We see Chuck Hildreth, another research subject for DEKA who lost both arms at eighteen in an electrical accident, remove a grape from its vine and bring it to his mouth. For the first time in nearly thirty years he is able to pick up an object by hand. A vibrating sensor allows the men to feel how tightly they are grasping things. "The feeling," Downs says, "is hard to describe. But for the first time in forty years my left hand did this [illustrating with his right hand the action of grasping and making a fist]. I just choked up right now. It was an amazing feeling. I was twenty-three years old the last time I did that. It felt so good to move my arm again, to do things with it. Not as fast. But it worked!"

Pelley remarks, "You just said you could move 'my arm again.' Did it feel like your arm?"

Downs, nodding, replies, "It did. It did. It felt like my arm. It was me." We witness prosthetized rebirth.

The *60 Minutes* segment ends with a young biomechanical engineer at Duke University. Jonathan Kuniholm lost his arm in a roadside blast while serving as a marine reservist captain in Iraq. He calmly explains how he is imagining performing movements while also moving the muscles that remain in his arm. His muscles, in turn, send electrical impulses that are detected with the electrodes that are attached to the stump just below his elbow. The technique is based on a myoelectric sensor that uses a software program to connect nerves and muscles. Pelley, holding the DEKA Arm attached to Kuniholm's stump, asks him to imagine closing his hand. The DEKA hand flexes. "How much training is required to move this hand with those muscles? How long did it take you to learn how to do this?"

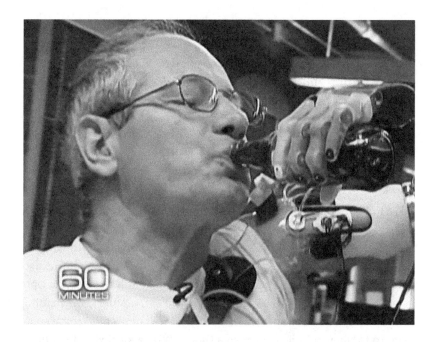

Kuniholm evenly responds, "I'm not really learning so much as the computer is. I'm doing what I imag-

FIG 3.9 / Fred Downs. From "The Pentagon's Bionic Arm," 60 Minutes, 2009.

ine I would like to do and we've taught the computer to interpret the signals [similar to the way a voice simulator is taught to speak words] and do what it takes [to perform the activity]."

"So it almost feels natural to you?" Pelley follows up.

"It does," Kuniholm responds.

I will return to the significance of this encounter between Pelley and Kuniholm in a few pages.

The segment concludes as Pelley qualifies that "after four years and $100 million, arms that can be controlled by thought are still a work in progress. But in the meantime, the DEKA Arm is now undergoing clinical testing at the VA in the hope that it will soon be available to the nearly 200 arm amputees from Iraq and Afghanistan." He means U.S. military service members, not the many thousands of civilians injured in those regions. Ling has the last word after Pelley asks him about the $100 million price tag for the research thus far: "It's a huge number. But it does a number of things. Number one of course, it fulfills our commitment to these fine young men and women who the issue of money compared to what they have done in service to the nation becomes immaterial. However, this is not a classified military weapons system [referring to much of what DARPA produces]. This is an advancement in medical technology. And the beauty of this particular effort is that this is another gift of the American taxpayer to the entire world." The familiar logic of debt owed to those who served and redemption through technoscientific salvation is enhanced by the imperial gesture of benefiting the world.

SELLING ARMS AT TED

Todd Kuiken, whose targeted muscle reinnervation technique I discussed earlier, was eager to advance the field of upper-limb prosthetics design, hoping to figure out a way to connect the devices directly to the human nervous system. Affiliated with the Rehabilitation Institute of Chicago (RIC) and the Biomedical Engineering Department at Northwestern University, Kuiken referred to himself as a physiatrist, capturing his training as both a physician and an engineer. Others called him a biomedical engineer. In October 2011 he presented a Global TED Talk titled "A Prosthetic Arm That 'Feels.'" Performing a ritual TED Talk secular circumambulation, the scientist moves around the stage under projected photographs of arm amputee patients, including one of a soldier in uniform and several others of adults and children with "Motivation" as the slide's title. He tells the audience that his motivation for working on upper-limb prosthetics is the reality that arm amputation causes a "huge disability" of multiple dimensions: not only does it make daily functioning difficult, but it also has a profound social and emotional impact. Gesticulating, he continues, "We talk with our hands, we greet with our hands, we interact with the physical world with our hands. To lose a hand or both hands is to lose these social capabilities." The stage is set for the dramatization of transcendent hybridization that Cassandra Crawford theorized, in which a hegemonic ableism centrally operates.

Kuiken rehearses the commonplace that prosthetic science for upper-body limbs lags behind that for lower limbs. He complains that for amputees above the elbow, the new neural-controlled devices are sometimes useless because there is not enough supportive muscle to operate the devices.[65] To address the deficit, Kuiken's team at RIC built an arm that added some wrist action and shoulder movement to get up to six degrees of freedom, using six motors. The team's aspirations were much greater: they wanted to develop a "neural interface, a way to our nervous system or to our thought processes so that it [the prosthetic arm and its movements] is intuitive." What was needed, in other words, was a signaling system that mimics how the healthy neural-limb interface works.

Offering a basic primer on the nervous system, Kuiken describes it as a communication system, whereby motor commands that originate in the brain are able to travel down the spinal cord and into the peripheral nerves in order to get the body to do something. The same system works in reverse: sensations derived from touching something (or smelling, hearing, seeing, or tasting something) travel back up the nerves and the spinal cord to the brain. Kuiken's solution was to develop the technique of targeted reinnervation, using the nervous system that persists following an amputation (previously attributed to sensations of "ghost limbs") to produce a "biological amplifier" that could amplify the nerve signals that go back and forth between the brain and the prosthetic limb via the spinal cord and "orphan" nerves.

The procedure, however, is significantly invasive, as illustrated in the case of Jesse Sullivan, the first man Kuiken's team treated. Sullivan was a fifty-four-year-old electrical lineman when he touched the wrong wire and was electrocuted with 7,200 volts. At the time of the accident in May 2001, he was so severely burned that he had to have both arms amputated up to the shoulder. The RIC originally fitted him with regular prostheses that attached to his torso and that he could control using buttons placed near his chin. As it happened, Sullivan required some "revision surgery" on his chest related to his injury; as Kuiken told the story, "that gave the medical team an opportunity to do targeted reinnervation." The surgery consisted of cutting away the nerves to Sullivan's muscle, then taking the arm nerves and shifting them down into his chest. The surgical team also inserted three electrodes to record signals that would become the syntax of imagined movements and sensations to program the signaling microprocessor later. With Sullivan's nerve endings of his arms surgically embedded in his chest, the nerves grew gradually so that after about three months, the researchers were able to "get a twitch" of the nerves' impulse. After six months it was actually possible for the researchers and Sullivan to see strong contractions under the skin of each of his breasts. After considerable physical therapy, he was able to move toy blocks from one location to another faster with the new myoelectrical limb. After several more months he was able to feel his hand when he was touched at a certain location on the chest where the nerve endings had been reinnervated. He reported being able to feel cold and hot, sharp and dull sensations and to sense his pinky and other fingers when a little pressure was placed on the relocated nerve endings.

Kuiken's TED talk included a demonstration with another "research collaborator," Amanda Kitts, a middle-aged white woman who lost an arm in a 2006 car accident. She had the targeted reinnervation surgery and in the next six months learned how to use her thoughts to control her arm and her elbow simultaneously. Kitts and Sullivan are among more than fifty patients worldwide on whom Kuiken had performed reinnervation surgery by 2011, about a dozen of them military veterans. He reported a 96 percent success rate. But in his effort to provide prostheses users with greater degrees of hand and arm freedom, he ran into "a real estate problem": there wasn't enough space on any patient's chest to attach the necessary number of electrodes to achieve more freedom of motion, a design challenge for the future. Another design problem was that prosthetic arms were made for the fiftieth-percentile (average) male body, making the devices too big for five-eighths of the world. Kuiken announced that the next arm his team would build would be designed for "the twenty-fifth percentile female body," which would also presumably fit a greater percentage of men's bodies in the world. The device would have a hand that can clasp, open all the way, and have two degrees of freedom in the wrist and elbow. It would also be "the smallest, the lightest, and the smartest arm ever made."

Kuiken concluded the TED Talk by recounting "the dark side" of this technology. If the audience thought this meant he would talk about ethical questions about the use of bionics, for example as militarized robots for use in combat, or about the exponential cost of the technology, they must have been surprised when he referred to the unpredictable behavior of such high-tech devices. He described Kitts arriving at the TED conference, jet-lagged, and putting on the arm: "Everything goes wrong. There was a computer spook, a broken wire, a computer that sparked. We took out a whole circuit in the hotel and just about put out the fire alarm." If it weren't for his highly qualified research team, who actually fixed the arm, he wouldn't have been able to demonstrate it for the audience. "That's science," he quipped, gesturing toward Kitts, "and fortunately it worked today." The audience gave him a standing ovation.

A DISSENTING VOICE

Despite his seeming endorsement of the DEKA Arm during his interview with Pelley, Kuniholm later had a story to tell that problematized the technological salvation message of the *60 Minutes* segment on upper-limb prosthetics. A little background on Kuniholm is useful here. He joined the marines in 1997 at the age of twenty-four and served on active duty for three and a half years, then entered a graduate program in industrial design at North Carolina State University. A few years later he was accepted into the PhD program in biomedical engineering at Duke University. While a graduate student, in 2004 he joined a Marine Reserve unit out of Lynchburg, Virginia. By that time he had started a company to build a robot that was able to move ahead of a patrol and defuse bombs before they exploded. But that venture was put on hold when, within forty-eight hours after joining the reserve unit, he received orders to deploy to Anwar Province in Iraq, where he was to serve as his unit's engineer. Four months after he arrived the thirty-three-old captain was searching for hidden bombs following an insurgent ambush of his unit near Haditha. Suddenly he was blasted off his feet by a bomb that was hidden in an olive oil can. While insurgents fired on his unit, he looked for his rifle and discovered that it was destroyed in the bomb blast. Then he realized that his right forearm was hanging by a thin strip of flesh from the rest of his arm. He grabbed his severed right hand and ran for cover. He was evacuated to a field hospital, where his arm was amputated, and then airlifted to Germany for medical treatment before being transported back to Duke University for surgery. Following all this he was sent to Walter Reed, where he received two prosthetic arms. One was a body-operated Dorrance model, patented in 1912, with a hook that opened and closed. The other was a myloelectric arm that he later described as heavy and limited in function, with electrodes embedded in its sleeve that picked up signals from the residual muscle in his forearm. The device was so heavy and awkward that he found himself using the older hook device instead. In this way he was not unlike the 90 percent of all arm amputees who wear prosthetics. Only 5 percent of this group wears an electronic prosthesis. Over 50 percent of all arm amputees abandon their devices because of awkwardness or discomfort. This state of affairs troubled Kuniholm.

As with Hugh Herr, Kuniholm's amputation and the limitations of existing prosthetic technology prompted him to direct the efforts of his

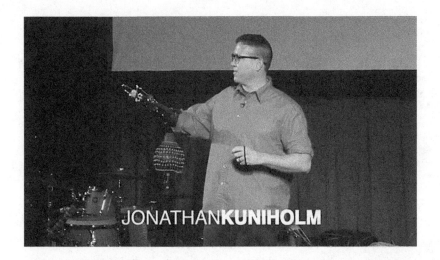

JONATHAN**KUNIHOLM**

company, Tackle Design, based in Dur-   FIG 3.10 / Jonathan Kuniholm giving
ham, North Carolina, to make better   his TEDx Talk.
prosthetics. But in contrast to Herr,
Kuniholm was less dazzled by neural prosthetics and the idea of building
a brain-machine interface; it seemed to him to be invasive and impracti-
cal, and it would be too expensive for most amputees to afford. In a 2009
interview with National Public Radio, around the time of the 60 Minutes
segment, he pointed out that myloelectric arms were too heavy and too
difficult to attach to the body to function well.[66] In a 2011 TEDx Talk he
recalled that he "spent half the day telling 60 Minutes that the real story was
about the economics of providing arms and what we got was a minute and
a half of 'gee whiz, thought-controlled arm.' And that's something that is
very distressing to me. The story is complicated. It's not a disaster. We are
doing the best we can. But what we have to put on people is simply not as
good as we think it is."

As an engineer he was irked that the device broke down often and was
less functional than the old Dorrance hook-and-stick device from 1912. He
complained that, because they were classified as cosmetic devices by most
insurance companies, they were too costly for most amputees to afford.
Some insurance policies covered prosthetic devices but with lifetime caps as
low as $1,500. The higher-tech prototype devices started at around $35,000
and ranged up to over $300,000 apiece. Kuniholm was also irritated by the
politics of government funding for research. He complained that DARPA
funding for prosthetics science and design, while substantial, was not even

a fraction of what was spent by the federal government for research and development of weapons systems. The government's priorities seemed out of whack to him. He also was frustrated that scientists would apply for grants in areas that were hot—such as neural bionics—even if the devices they were developing were not what amputees wanted or needed. He criticized university-based engineers and scientists who "offered solutions in search of problems," eager to get their hands on government money that could be spent on more practical devices. Private industry, in his view, was also to blame since much more money was invested in makers of video game hardware and software (with annual industry sales of $17 billion in 2010) and erectile dysfunction drugs ($3–4 billion in 2010) than was invested in electronic arms. The upper-limb amputee population was, Kuniholm said, "an underserved population." Furthermore, while military veterans had their prosthetic devices paid for by the government, they constituted a very small percentage of the population of people missing arms in the United States. From 2003 to 2011, 186 military members lost part of an arm, while around 70,000 in the civilian population were missing parts of an arm. And millions around the world have lost arms as a consequence of war-related activities, a reality Kuniholm did not mention. But he worried that the promoters of high-tech prosthetics failed to address the problem of who would have access to them.[67]

As a disabled person, Kuniholm calls out the "two-armed bias" that manifests in designers' preoccupation with how prosthetic arms look. "If you ask most amputees, what they really want is to restore functionality and not how realistic the hand might look. There are a lot of sacrifices that end up being made in trying to make something look like a hand and so a lot of people look at these hooks and their first reaction is 'gosh, I wouldn't want to walk around with that thing attached to me.' . . . I think that a lot of prosthetics have been designed by the two-handed and to make the two-handed feel better."[68] He worries about pie-in-the-sky schemes that play well as media stories but fail to serve the most pressing needs of amputees. He does not want to wait around for "thought-controlled" prosthetics or submit himself to "a clinical study that involves plugging things into my brain." Referring to the cultural afterlife of television's *Six Million Dollar Man*, he argues that "the $6 million meme . . . an idea that travels very quickly virally, that resonates with people and is capable of spreading . . . leaves the impression that thought-controlled arms are here and that we have kicked this problem when in fact we have not."

Prosthetics designers, in Kuniholm's view, need to spend more time talking with amputees about their needs and what will best benefit them rather than designing devices that are not practical and that almost no one can afford. He criticizes private companies that are funded by taxpayers' money to do prosthetics research and are granted the right to hold a monopoly over what they develop, at least for some period of time, rather than sharing it with others. To address these concerns, Kuniholm cofounded the Open Prosthetics Project: An Initiative of the Shared Design Alliance, an open-source collaboration between designers, users, and funders with hundreds of members from around the world. The project's tagline is "Prosthetics Shouldn't Cost an Arm and a Leg."[69] Its mission is to foster the making of prosthetic designs and to share information for anyone to use and build on. It was set up as a social media platform. Kuniholm's blog entries discuss the everyday experiences of using prosthetic arms and the design challenges that need to be addressed. Written in lay terms, they offer advice to readers and caution them to be wary of the hype of some prosthetic scientists and companies.

Kuniholm was one of four veterans chosen to speak at the 2008 Democratic National Convention in Denver, where he endorsed Obama while criticizing Republican nominee John McCain's support for the war in Iraq, a war that he said "was a bad idea and poorly planned at the highest levels."[70] On the issue of government funding for scientific projects, Kuniholm shares the Obama administration's subsequent endorsement of public-private partnerships for funding scientific research. He likens his open-source platform to the funding that went into all of the advances in prosthetics design following World War II, when the U.S. government held the resulting patents. Privately held patents and intellectual property restrictions stall scientific advancement, in his view. At the same time he acknowledges that private investment can be useful for stimulating a competitive edge and getting products to market. He worries, however, that private corporations are not following through on manufacturing affordable products that are useful to those who most need them. In other words, they are taking public funding but failing to develop or serve the market. His goal of starting a company that is majority-owned by service-disabled veterans who have "skin in the game" is faithful to the tenets of entrepreneurial innovation that typify politically progressive tech startup companies.

Though Kuniholm is clearly invested in running a successful business, his preference for open-source information sharing and his emphasis on making products that people can actually use resonate with the not-for-profit Science for the People movement that grew out of the antiwar and free speech movements of the 1960s. Scientists and engineers active in the nonprofit community-based Science Shops argue for ethical scientific practices and advocate for research and critical dialogue that will further the kind of knowledge and inventions that will improve rather than endanger or limit people's lives. It is a movement to democratize science. A central concern is exposing how science is misused to support unequal social relations, including the profit-driven privatization of publicly funded research and the war-profiteering of weapons scientists. In 2014 a group at MIT began an effort to revive the movement and focused on increasing demographic diversity within the STEM professions while also advocating open discussions of the ethical, social, and political consequences of science and technology. Like this revival, Kuniholm's dissenting voice and his organizing through the Open Prosthetics Project offer the possibility for disentangling some of the life-limiting attachments to war that are nestled in what I have been calling biomedical salvation narratives.

SYNOPSIS

This chapter has focused on advanced bionic devices as they signify a cultural enchantment with the idea of bodily enhancement. Their charismatic inventors describe these new devices as repayments of debt owed to soldiers injured in war and citizens injured in domestic terrorist attacks. Blending elements of performance art, athletics, and choreography, they shift the focus away from bed-ridden suffering and toward aesthetic performances that dramatize how injuries can be overcome and nature's limits exceeded. Hope and optimism are central to their narratives of bionic enhancement. Recovering patients are praised for their adaptability, determination, and hard work, character traits that are valorized in physical rehabilitation as an allegory of national rehabilitation in the context of war-weariness and the persistent worry of terrorist attacks in the homeland.

The spectacle of veterans being fitted with neural bionics is commonly presented as a kind of prosthetic rebirth through which the injured person, if he or she works hard enough, can become "better than ever." The able among us are reminded that we owe a debt to those whose injuries are propelling technoscience forward. As prostheses attach their wearers to war, they attach many more of us to biomedical devices through fantasies of superhuman ability. Publicity about bionic assemblages, from TED Talks and *60 Minutes* to *Wired* magazine, connect consumerist interest in fitness culture and makeovers with computational robotics through tropes of self-mastery, overcoming odds, and striving for perfection. Technology is made to appear compassionate, bold, and ever-improving. Fashioning one's body in the accounts I have related is tied to fulfilling the self. Regimes of rehabilitation and adaptation to bionic devices are animated with a kind of technoscientific faith healing in which great hope is invested in what these feats of engineering can do for us all.

The war-wounded veteran who has survived a near-death experience is the subject of hyperhabilitation so long as he or she exhibits a willingness to embrace the new device. A politics of visibility is notable here. Rehabilitation is as much a performance to be witnessed as a process for the patient to go through. Rather than being sequestered out of public view, the veteran in rehabilitative therapy should be seen. The affective economy of sympathy infuses this demand for visibility and draws the witness close to the patient who is learning to walk, touch, or feel again. What great satisfaction the witness should feel when watching the dedicated patient work hard to become independent again. What a relief. What an avenue for salvation. These are the feelings that the media productions I have discussed in this chapter valorize.

Twenty-first-century prosthetics science reflects the affective disposition required to be able to cope with post-Fordist flexible capitalism, where uncertainty is one of the few constants. The ideal person is encouraged to be agile, to have physical stamina, to play well on a team, but also to take responsibility for his or her own failings. He or she must take risks and be ready to change quickly. Self-improvement, biomedical salvation, care, and beneficence suffuse the world of TED Talks and *60 Minutes* presentations on neural bionics. The secular priesthood offering these gifts includes scientists and engineers who may seem well-meaning. They belong to a creative class of the up-and-coming and the arrived who, far from fitting the stereotype of the detached scientist or asocial engineer, express their patriotism by attending to those damaged in war.

Neural bionic devices are expensive and functionally deficient. Who is worthy of enhancement? Who is not? The *60 Minutes* segments on rehabilitation featured patients who were wounded in war or in vehicular accidents. Missing were people whose amputations resulted from diabetes or other conditions that are medically manageable if the sufferers had access to health insurance and good medical care. Also missing from the feature stories were any of the thousands of Afghans and Iraqis who lost limbs during the U.S. invasion and occupation of their countries. The yawning divide between high-tech bionics therapies available to a relatively few in the United States and the almost nonexistent medical care in the regions the United States and its coalition allies invaded lays bare the profoundly limited promises of bionic enhancement.

FOUR

Pathogenic Threats

On Pharmaceutical War Profiteering

On September 29, 2005, the last day of the fiscal year, when Congress was supposed to complete its budgeting process for the next year, a group of Democratic senators, led by Tom Harkin (Iowa), introduced an amendment to the FY 2006 Defense Appropriations bill.[1] It would dedicate $3 billion to preparing for the imminent arrival of the avian influenza H5N1 virus to the United States. A hearing the senators attended the day before with the heads of the CDC and the NIH warned that the nation's public health infrastructure would be overwhelmed when the flu hit the United States. Harkin, Ted Kennedy, and Barack Obama, then a junior senator from Illinois, argued before the Senate that the amendment was urgently needed. In their view the federal government had fumbled badly when it was not prepared for the attacks on September 11 or for Hurricane Katrina, which had devastated New Orleans just weeks earlier. The hearing with the CDC and NIH was a lobbying effort to counter the Bush administration's proposed cuts of $133 million from the CDC and $33 million from public health funding for hospital preparedness.

A bellicose Ted Stevens, Republican from Alaska, initially opposed the amendment, doubting that avian flu could be transmitted between humans and arguing that the amendment should not be attached to the defense budget. He was adamant that troops serving in Iraq and Afghanistan had more important needs. Stevens added that if Harkin wanted legislation for avian flu preparedness, the amendment should be addressed to the Health and Human Services budget. "But we don't have time to go through that process," Harkin protested. "Tomorrow is the last day for making amendments to appropriations bills. And when it comes to the outbreak of avian flu in the United States, it is not a matter of *if* but *when!*" The Democratic senators provided charts showing that the H5N1 virus had already sickened many humans, birds, and mammals in Southeast Asia and Hong Kong and had a fatality rate of 50 percent in humans. In typical fashion, last-minute quarrels over annual budget appropriations featured senators invoking urgency as a rhetorical tool to support their budgetary goals. Citing the nation's defense is a common tactic in this annual ritual.

Amid the bickering, Richard Burr, a five-term U.S. representative and in 2005 a newly elected Republican senator from North Carolina, spoke calmly in sympathy with Harkin's amendment but proposed what he called a more comprehensive approach to emergency preparedness for pandemic disease. As head of the subcommittee on bioterrorism, Burr had been holding hearings that informed his plan to write legislation that would fulfill the CDC's Strategic National Stockpile, mandated by Congress in 1999 to store vaccines and other "medical countermeasures" in the event of a public health emergency. Harkin commended Burr for his idea but stressed that there was no time to delay. Fellow Democrats argued for the amendment's inclusion in the defense budget because avian flu, while not a recognized bioterrorist weapon, would bring war to the United States and the enemy would be an influenza virus. The country was spending $2 billion each week on the war in Iraq, and the president's proposed budget for defense was $442 billion for 2006; surely, they argued, the American people deserved to be protected against biological threats, and the meager 1 million available doses of flu vaccine would leave the vast majority at risk.

As a tactic to restore funding to the CDC and NIH, the senators framed medical preparedness in terms of defense against an enemy virus in what they argued would be an inevitable war with influenza. "Quite frankly," Harkin insisted, "this is about defense. It is about defending our people—not against a terrorist but against terrorism, the terrorism of an avian flu pandemic."[2]

To make sense of Burr's position, it helps to go back a few years earlier, when deadly pathogens were sent through the U.S. mail just weeks after September 11, 2001. Five letters laced with anthrax spores were mailed to two U.S. Democratic senators and various media outlets. Five people who handled the mail died and seventeen became ill in what the FBI referred to as the worst biological attacks in U.S. history. The FBI and its partners began an investigation code-named *Amerithrax*, a strange linguistic blending that fused *America* with *anthrax* in what was about to become the massive expansion of the emerging counterterror state. Between 2001 and 2008 the investigation gathered more than ten thousand witness interviews on six continents and issued over five thousand grand jury subpoenas, along with collecting thousands of environmental samples from sixty different locations.[3]

This chapter offers an account of how biomedical logics operated in the vast expansion of research related to biological threats that took place during the first decades of the twenty-first century, a time marked by growing anxiety about the likelihood of future bioterrorist attacks. I will examine the consequences of the domestic anthrax scare of 2001 in terms of attaching ordinary people to the apparatus of counterterrorism funded by tax payers and fueled by the sentiment of fear. I will discuss developments from the 1990s in order to show why, by 2014, pharmaceutical manufacturers had profited handsomely from government contracts leading up to and after Bush's announcement of the Global War on Terror. I argue that biotechnology and pharmaceutical companies, along with the elected officials they lobbied, exploited the emotions of dread and suspicion enabled by the massive expansion of the counterterror state that spurred an unprecedented surge in biomedical war profiteering. Whereas hope was the central affect of regenerative medicine and bionic prosthetics research, the negative emotion of insecurity saturates the discourse and practices of the counterterror state and the biomedical countermeasures industry it supported. Manufacturers and their advocates in government emphasized the dangers of viruses and other pathogens as existential threats while saying little about how their own research practices and novel products heightened the risks associated with biological weapons of mass destruction. In fact the structured silence on industry-generated dangers worked to fuel product demand: pathogenic risks, whatever their origins, promised an expanding market for bioengineered commodities and increased the appeal of otherwise flagging biotechnology stock portfolios. Meanwhile widespread cultural suspicion about the government's role in poisoning the population with bioweapons experimentation attached ordinary people to war in deeply discomforting ways. What could be done about the government's denial of responsibility for Persian Gulf War veterans suffering from debilitating illnesses after receiving mandated vaccines? What were we to do about the news that a demented government researcher was sending anthrax spores with scrawled threats through the mail to news anchors, members of Congress, and even a sorority house? How were ordinary people to make sense of verified revelations of Cold War–era secret pathogenic experiments on domestic populations? Bioweapons research has ghoulish, dystopic undertones. It exists in a narrative framework inflected with mistrust, paranoia, and conspiracy.

The longer history of modern disease intervention in the United States is rife with racialized fantasies of infection perpetrated by "outsiders"— immigrants, guest workers, traders, sex workers, "degenerates," and the colonized. In its continental and more recent planetary reach, U.S. empire, as Neel Ahuja has argued, has been preoccupied by fantasies of the dangers that come with military, economic, and territorial expansion for over a century. "The forces of imperial disease intervention," Ahuja writes, "constituted settler bodies and ecologies as an emergent space of technocratic control, rendering them lively domains of warfare."[4] Preventing transmission of disease across borders and establishing surveillance systems for tracking and quarantining manifest the logic of imperial disease intervention. While staging itself as universally valuable to the whole of society in the form of public health, this form of disease intervention exposed its partiality through the circulation of racial fears of disease. Disease interventions dating from the early years of the twentieth century were modeled on territorial warfare in which bodies were to be sorted—some defended and others vanquished. Epidemiology as a form of biopolitical governance transformed biological processes into sites of surveillance and population management. The racialization of transborder pandemics intensified anti-foreigner xenophobia while also generating public faith in the imperial state as a vigilant guardian of life and the free market as an efficient means for controlling disease.

The 2006 Senate debate over funding to prepare for the imminent arrival of the H5N1 virus from overseas reflected this longer history of imperial disease control in which fantasies of control target some bodies for state intervention in the name of national security.[5] By the time the Senate debated funding for H5N1 detection, new boundaries of an older racialized cordon sanitaire had been drawn around the figures of the infected migrant and the terrorist with weapons of mass destruction. What emerged in the early years of the twenty-first century was a sense that, in an age of globalization, existential threats were potentially everywhere. The official concern was that these threats were constantly evolving. They could be activated either accidentally or intentionally. Their rapid mutation compounded the challenge of disease detection and control. The ability to genetically modify organisms in laboratories added to the worry that "emergent" threats required an anticipatory apparatus. This thinking authorized the massive expansion of the U.S. national security state with an unprecedented investment in biosecurity, a set of practices aimed at protecting human health and protecting agricultural produce through the prevention, control, and management of biological risk factors. Following the anthrax attacks of 2001, the emergent counterterror state amplified these practices by anticipating acts of intentional bioterrorism. Along with the emergence of this counterterror state came new profit-making opportunities for private contractors pitching biosecurity products.

THE ANTHRAX LETTERS AND A
RENEWED SECURITY STATE

Even more than the suicide-hijacker attacks of 9/11, the anthrax letters enabled the American national security apparatus to, as Joseph Masco has observed, "renew itself in the twenty-first century, replacing the nuclear weapons-centered vision of the twentieth-century national security state with the 'terrorist with a WMD [weapon(s) of mass destruction]' fixation of the counterterror state." The letters unleashed an official concern that existing government agencies were not prepared for dealing with biological attacks. Masco persuasively argues that, in their wake, a new concept of American power emerged that is founded on a "radical and never-ending insecurity, whose objects multiply to the point where the only territorial limit to U.S. defense is the entire planet." Securing life on a global scale became a goal of domestic defense. Seeing the world as full of uncertainties and existential threats that take infinite forms, the American counterterror state was the creation of "hyperpower geopolitics, affectively driven governance, and deep multigenerational commitment to militarization." It is a world-making project afflicted by a mood of pessimism, fatalism, and menace, "one structured at every level by apocalyptic intuitions and commitments."[6]

The mass disruption caused by the anthrax letters revealed that the nation was vulnerable to multiple forms of terrorism. A specific concern for controlling anthrax morphed into the larger threat of WMD in the Bush administration's discourse on terrorism. As national security expanded to planetary security, the ties between war and public health deepened. The terrorist, WMD, and the pathogen became fused together. Each was subject to evolving definitions. This made the existential threat they presented all the more politically and affectively powerful. The counterterror state exploited this free-floating anxiety to do many things. One was to justify invading Iraq. Holding a small vial of simulated anthrax, Secretary of State Colin Powell famously testified before the United Nations in February 2003 that Saddam Hussein had weapons of mass destruction.[7] The vial contained less than a teaspoon of powder. Powell told the assembly that it was about the amount of what had been sent in the anthrax envelopes that shut down the U.S. Senate in the fall of 2001. He cited a UN Special Commission's estimate that Hussein had the ability to produce up to 25,000 liters of anthrax, which "if concentrated into this dry form would be enough to fill tens upon tens upon tens of thousands of teaspoons." On these grounds the Bush administration made the case for preemptive war. Fear, anger, and paranoia were strategic elements in their arsenal.

Another outcome of the anthrax letters scare was the massive expansion of the "homeland security" apparatus into which billions of dollars were poured. In the name of biodefense, federal funding for biotechnology, pharmaceutical products, and disease surveillance systems increased substantially, opening up a new channel of war profiteering for private contractors in these industries. In his 2003 State of the Union speech Bush proposed that $6 billion be earmarked "to quickly make available effective vaccines and treatments against agents like anthrax, botulinum toxin, Ebola, and plague. We must assume that our enemies would use these as weapons, and we must act before the dangers are upon us."[8] Within months of Bush's speech Congress authorized $5.593 billion under a new program called Project BioShield to purchase vaccines and fund research on medical countermeasures against what were assumed to be imminent or emergent biological attacks. By the time the Senate was arguing over funding for avian flu preparedness in 2005, Richard Burr, representing a state with strong biotechnology and pharmaceutical industries, saw a need and an opportunity to legislate something much bigger.[9] The result was passage of the Pandemic and All-Hazard Preparedness legislation in 2006, which established the Biological Advanced Research and Development Authority (BARDA) and expanded the sprawling labyrinth of biosecurity agencies that sprang up in response to the anthrax bioterrorist attacks of 2001. These initiatives opened the floodgates for tax money to be awarded to private pharmaceutical companies who retooled their operations to prepare for war at home. A Republican majority in the Congress and the Bush administration were intent on diverting funding previously dedicated to the nation's public health infrastructure toward private contractors specializing in biotechnology and pharmaceutical production.

As Global War on Terror rhetoric put emphasis on biological threats, the disciplines of public health, microbiology, and genetic engineering became entangled with war in new ways. In the scenario of twenty-first-century biological warfare, the battlefield is not in some distant locale and the enemy need not be a person. Pathogenic war is instead characterized as ubiquitous, a menace that is indifferent to national boundaries and that may be microscopic. A "homegrown terrorist" could unleash this kind of war. So could an unwitting traveler infected with a virus or a child whose parents refuse to vaccinate her. The emerging market for biotechnological security was fueled by a dreadful and urgent sense of ever-intensifying risk. The industry was oriented toward anticipating what Secretary of Defense Rumsfeld referred to as "known unknowns"—threats that loomed but whose specific biological qualities required expensive research in order to detect, prevent, contain, or therapeutically treat them.[10] In this anticipatory mind-set, the future invades the present and takes it hostage by predicting risks and speculating on novel drugs and engineering mutated pathogens, some of which posed considerable biological risks.[11] Speculation involves considerable risk not just in financial markets but also in laboratory practices that produce more virulent biological agents in the name of gaining mastery over them. Panic excites new waves of biological weapons research. Our own scientists engineered new dangers in the name of countering them, even as surveillance devices produced false positives and otherwise unpredicted disease outbreaks surfaced. Containment is a fading fantasy. At the same time pharmaceutical marketing campaigns stress the need for faith in "forward-looking therapies" and brand slogans that pair biosecurity with life enhancement. These are the conditions of possibility that deepen the historically extensive attachments of the pharmaceutical industry to war and expand these attachments more overtly to dreams of exploiting recombinant DNA technology to fight wars at the molecular level. Terror attaches an anxious public to the promises these industries offer via congressional authorizations of vast sums of money given to a handful of private companies contracted for the purposes of replenishing the alarmingly insufficient Strategic National Stockpile of medical countermeasures to disease outbreaks.

In previous chapters I explored the dynamic relationship of indebtedness that rationalized war as necessary for technosalvation, with the soldier's injured body as a central figure in the narrative of redemption and expiation. Care and benevolence toward the ailing patient were central tropes in the logics at play in the biomedical salvation narrative. Here we confront a situation in which the bodies of soldiers are not ultimately exceptional. An ethic of care is mitigated by nervous anticipation that outbreaks loom all around. In the face of imminent and emergent threats, all bodies are conceived as potentially threatened or threatening, and some more threatening than others. People become attached to war through terror of being quietly and covertly put at risk at the micro level by new and more virulent mutating germs, viruses, and toxins, whether by intentional acts or accidental exposure. Bodies are in this sense both potentially targets and weapons—victims and vectors—in the apocalyptic framing of ominous doom. As Stefan Elbe has noted, citizens are conceived, as they have been in past public health emergencies, as potential agents of disease with a sense of impending emergency.[12] Triage procedures resonate with racial profiling. Some bodies become sites of covert experimentation in the name of protecting others. National insecurity is framed as an urgent medical problem dramatized by an enemy attacking the inner workings of vulnerable human organisms in the scary form of "silent killers." Medical professionals are mobilized to do the security work of detection, contact tracing, and quarantining while also being enlisted to conduct research that promises to result in effective antidotes and preventative vaccines. Whereas modern war has often been translated as an allegory of medical intervention, as we saw in the way counterinsurgency operations are conceived, in biowarfare and biosecurity the allegory is replaced by a definition of war as itself a matter of medical intervention. The war is waged on, through, and with microscopic pathogens. A politics of life in which biological systems must be fortified against attacks exists amid the specter of undetected and latent deadly agents capable of mass destruction. For biosecurity companies, panic is a useful marketing tool.

GOING PLANETARY: GLOBAL HEALTH SECURITY IN THE AGE OF COUNTERTERRORISM

Prior to 2001 biosecurity was generally defined in veterinary science as a practice for preventing the spread of disease among livestock and crops, using techniques of isolation, traffic control, and sanitation to be applied on farms. The shift from a focus on livestock and crop security to include terrorist attacks as well as naturally occurring outbreaks and then to encompass emergent biological threats created new opportunities for alliances across health, drug, and defense institutions, attaching the nation to war through an affective state of perpetual anxiety and preparedness. Since one can never have too much health or too much security, the biosecurity apparatus of the United States has expanded to a planetary scale. The CDC, for example, operates on military bases overseas in Africa, Latin America, and Southeast Asia, seeking to detect and control threats that may jump species from animals to humans. CDC efforts there are aimed, in part, at preventing infected bodies from entering the United States.[13]

The planetary reach of U.S. biosecurity initiatives can be seen as part of a larger trend toward what Andrew Lakoff has called the regime of global health security.[14] This formation focuses on emerging infectious diseases that are assumed to pose a threat to wealthy nations and are identified as originating in Latin America, sub-Saharan Africa, and parts of Asia. Most recently identified threats are avian influenza, smallpox, weaponized severe acute respiratory syndrome (SARS), and the Ebola and Zika viruses. Global health security is oriented toward threats that may not have happened yet or that may never happen. It focuses on preparedness to prevent or minimize the consequences of potentially devastating pandemics. It mobilizes national disease control institutes, laboratories, and multilateral health agencies, using disease surveillance methods, emergency operations centers, and vaccine distribution systems.

Global health security as such grew out of a series of developments in post–World War II world health governance. Since its inception in 1948, the World Health Organization has coordinated national public health agencies in order to promote disease eradication with vaccination campaigns. As a consequence of international human rights activism, arguing that health care was a basic human right, the WHO implemented primary health care in developing nations. But this primary care model fell into crisis in the early 1990s, when funds devoted to it dwindled as the World Bank, a principal funder of developing states, pivoted to reforming national health systems as part of its structural adjustment plans. Primary care was traded off in the World Bank's pressure on developing nations to pay back loans. Attempting to make up the difference, the WHO shifted its direction to public-private partnerships that focused on specific diseases, such as HIV/AIDS and tuberculosis. The Bill and Melinda Gates Foundation was a key player in this trend, granting $1.7 billion to projects in 1998–2000. The Clinton Global Initiative and the UN Global Fund followed. The shift, however, came at the expense of supporting local health infrastructures.

As Lakoff argues, the disease-focused philanthropic efforts of the Gates and Clinton foundations belong to a regime of humanitarian biomedicine, which he differentiates from the regime of global health security. While both are aimed at managing infectious disease on a global scale, "each regime rests on very different visions of both the social order that is at stake in global health and the most appropriate technical means for achieving it."[15] Humanitarian biomedicine targets diseases that afflict the poorer nations of the world, such as malaria, TB, and HIV/AIDS, and is usually applied where the local public health infrastructure is weak or nonexistent. Funders seek to bring advanced diagnostic and pharmaceutical interventions to those in need. They do so, in part, by stimulating the production of needed pharmaceutical products and biotechnology for serving people suffering from "neglected diseases."

Lakoff argues that while global health security focuses on prophylaxis against potential threats at home by demanding compliance from national governments elsewhere, humanitarian biomedicine "invests resources to mitigate present suffering in other places." Actors within each regime "work to craft a space of the global that will be a site of knowledge and intervention," but the regimes differ in the type of ethical relationship they assume between health care advocates and the afflicted. This relationship can be "one of either moral obligation to the other or protection against the risk to the self. Global health is, in this sense, a contested ethical, political, and technical zone whose contours are still under construction."[16] Because global health security regimes focus on detection, preparedness, and the protection of wealthy nations, the model is most closely aligned with the U.S. counterterror state's funding of biosecurity research, development, and implementation. Though they exist in some tension, alongside the counterterror state's investments in biosecurity are philanthropic initiatives to fund new pharmaceutical and biotechnological products. Thus both of these global health regimes contribute to disease- and war-related biomedical profiteering for private contractors.[17]

COUNTERMEASURES AND MUTUAL PROVOCATIONS

The case of biosecurity research brings to light a particular dynamic of mutual provocation between wounding and healing technologies, between infection and the production of medical knowledge. The term *medical countermeasure* itself signifies a mutual provocation between deleterious agents and the medical products designed to counter them. For nearly a century bioweapons research has been promoted not only as a strategy for defense but also as a means to advance knowledge in the fields of microbiology, immunology, infectious disease, genetics, and epidemiology.[18] Proponents argue that this knowledge can be applied to treat and prevent many health problems, not just those unleashed by biological attacks. War under these circumstances is redeemed in a particular way: by developing defenses against biological threats, life and scientific knowledge are purportedly improved. But the research itself has cost billions of dollars and carries substantial risks, particularly for communities and individuals upon whom clandestine experimentation has been conducted.

According to this logic, the nation's security is tied to its people's health and safety. In recent decades something called "globalization" has loomed as the condition of threats; as Angela Mitropoulos has observed, this "served to legitimate the depiction of nation-states as an organic entity."[19] Migration control has long been intertwined with public health in its quest to protect the body politic and enforce notions of proper nationalism. The disease-bearing migrant is demonized within this framework, as Priscilla Wald outlines in her analysis of Mary Mallon ("Typhoid Mary"), whose body signified a threat to both the destitute and the affluent, since typhoid afflicted both groups.[20] Mallon's body became a convenient means for warning of white "race suicide." At stake then and now is the national body's health and productivity, with tacit assumptions about which bodies pose threats. With the advent of globalization, the diseased migrant and the terrorist with WMD are seen as leading agents that put the nation's body at risk. Both are treated as suspicious and blameful, since the biosecurity apparatus of the counterterror state has blurred the distinction between accidental and intentional risk.

The distinction between offensive and defensive uses of biological weapons was previously a central tenet of international law that barred the former and permitted the latter in the name of research. It is moot in the context of preemptive war. For the purposes of laboratory research, distinguishing between intentional attacks and naturally occurring outbreaks makes little sense. In either case, as the logic goes, the nation will need a large stockpile of vaccines and antipathogen drugs. Gone too is the distinction between *imagined* and *real* threats. In the anticipatory logic of national defense that authorizes preemptive war, the nation must be ready for them all. A central problem for biodefense research is its dual-use quality: it can be helpful for learning how to prevent or treat outbreaks, and it can be used by individuals or groups seeking to do harm. The worry for biosecurity officials is that research on countermeasures and pathogens could be misapplied to cause destructive outcomes. This concern contributes to the mutual ratcheting up of bioweapons research on the one hand and an expanded security apparatus on the other. Indeed Dr. Anthony Fauci, head of the CDC, warned of the risks of biodefense research in the very same 2012 article in which he emphasized the funding opportunities offered by the counterterrorism apparatus.[21]

A review of the relevant historical context of biological weapons research helps to make sense of how military-funded research on pathogens enabled lobbyists for the biotechnology and pharmaceutical industries in the opening decade of the twenty-first century to take advantage of the permanent and pervasive nature of war now.

FROM A DOCTRINE OF DEFENSE TO THE
DOCTRINE OF COUNTERPROLIFERATION

International treaties dating back to the period following World War I outlawed the preemptive use of biological weapons but allowed laboratory research about them to be conducted in the name of defense. The 1925 Geneva Protocol that outlawed the use of biological weapons contained a provision allowing research on biological agents. The Protocol for the Prohibition of the Use in War of Asphyxiating, Poisonous or Other Gases, and of Bacteriological Methods of Warfare was signed at a conference held in Geneva in the summer of 1925 under the auspices of the League of Nations and went into effect in 1928. Regarded as a response to the extensive use and horrific suffering caused by chemical weapons during World War I, the 1925 Geneva Protocol called for a total ban on the development and use of chemical weapons. Only after Poland sought an amendment that would include bacterial weapons was the protocol amended to "extend this prohibition to the use of bacteriological methods of warfare."[22] France, which already had a developed biological weapons program, called for an exception; rather than complying with a total ban, the French demanded the right to develop weapons for the purpose of retaliation. This resulted in shifting the international rule from a total ban of chemical and biological weapons to a "no first use" policy. This exception to the original language allowed the United Kingdom and the Soviet Union to later justify their offensive programs in the name of defense while developing increasingly virulent and abundant stocks of deadly pathogens. The United States did not ratify the protocol until April 10, 1975.[23]

After World War II broke out, the U.S. Department of War responded by establishing a far-flung apparatus of federal research laboratories and facilities for stockpiling biological agents, coordinated with several leading pharmaceutical manufacturers. Similar to the Manhattan Project's development of nuclear bombs, American bioweapons research was rationalized from its inception as necessary to the nation's defense and carried out in secret. During the Cold War, researchers continued experimenting with pathogens and stockpiled biological agents in anticipation of a biological attack. Today much of the research on biodefense is conducted in for-profit company laboratories, less subject to the highly secretive strictures of the Cold War period and more to the demands of selling their wares as lifesaving substances. Centralized federal control is now offset by private companies seeking to attract investors.

In 1969, before much of the research was outsourced to private companies, President Richard Nixon, acting on advice from defense planners, renounced the government's biological weapons program on the grounds that germ warfare undermined the Cold War doctrine of mutual deterrence. He reasoned that pathogens were unpredictable and mobile and thus posed a danger to civilian populations at home and abroad. On April 10, 1972, the United States signed the Biological and Toxin Weapons Convention (BTWC), banning the use and possession of biological weapons. The measure was put into force in March 1975. But the BTWC did not ban biodefense research as long as it was dedicated to "prophylactic, protective, or other peaceful purposes."[24] Lacking sufficient enforcement, the BTWC did not put an end to bioweapons development and stockpiling in the United States or elsewhere. Proponents in the United States justified the continued research by arguing that the nation needed to know how to defend itself in case of a biological attack, and the only way to acquire knowledge about biological weapons was to experiment with producing and testing them. Most of the research and development was conducted in government laboratories at Fort Detrick, Maryland, and in other federally owned facilities around the United States.

When the Soviet Union dissolved in late 1991, American defense intellectuals speculated about military strategy in a post–Cold War world. Planners in the George H. W. Bush administration took an interest in the Revolution in Military Affairs, a hypothesis originally formulated in the 1970s and 1980s by Soviet commanders about the future of warfare in light of technological advancements and shifting geopolitics. As chief of the General Staff of the USSR Armed Forces from 1977 through 1984, Nikolai Vasilyevich Ogarkov oversaw the Soviet intervention in Afghanistan that began in late 1979. He sought to reduce the massive Soviet military to a smaller, more agile force that integrated advanced technology into its operations. As a loyal Communist Party member trained in engineering, he argued that nuclear warfare was intrinsically unstable and that this fact would give way to the development of new weapons and strategies, including the use of precision strikes, automated command and control, and electronic warfare.[25] Influenced by some of Ogarkov's ideas, hawkish strategists in the United States warned of a rise in terrorism and disruption generated by nonstate actors working in secretive networks aimed not at defending territory but at wreaking havoc. They cited biological warfare as one of the likely vectors of terrorism, pointing to a widely publicized case of biocrime from September 1984, when an obscure religious cult sought to gain influence in a local election in Oregon. Followers of Bhagwan Shree Rajneesh operated a medical laboratory in Antelope, Oregon, and purchased a bacterial strain of *Salmonella* from a commercial supplier in Seattle, which they cultivated and secretly distributed to salad bars at ten local restaurants so that people would be too sick to get to the polls. Over seven hundred people suffered from the food poisoning incident; forty-five were hospitalized, though none died. The cult had planned for a larger contamination of the local water supply after this trial run. The episode was devastating to the local economy. After a long investigation and prosecution process, the director of the Oregon State Public Health Laboratory commented, "The first significant biological attack on a U.S. community was not carried out by foreign terrorists smuggled into New York, but by legal residents of a U.S. community. The next time it happens it could be with more lethal agents. . . . We in public health are really not ready to deal with that."[26] U.S. military strategists argued for renewing the nation's investment in biological weapons research in the wake of this attack, coupled with their growing worry that scientists from the Soviet Union were migrating to Iraq and assisting in bioweapons development there.

Under President Bill Clinton, military strategists replaced the Cold War doctrine of mutual deterrence with the principle of counterproliferation. Whereas nonproliferation policy and arms control had been carried out by diplomatic, legal, and administrative measures to (in principle) prevent the development or acquisition of weapons of mass destruction, counterproliferation measures officially authorized military action and armed conflict to achieve these goals. In 1998 Clinton approved two new directives to improve the nation's ability to prevent and respond to biological attacks and appointed a veteran security expert, Richard Clarke, as the national coordinator for antiterrorism programs. Clinton designated the Environmental Protection Agency to assist the Departments of Justice and Defense in responding to threats.[27] His directives were supported by an additional $1 billion added to the defense budget for chemical and biological defense. The principle of counterproliferation in practice spurred the development of biowarfare agents rather than curtailing them.

The worry that belligerent regimes would use chemical and biological weapons in future conflicts provided the incentive for scaling up the manufacturing of countermeasures, particularly to deal with pathogens that had long been at the center of bioweapons research in U.S. laboratories. Chief among these was *Bacillus anthracis,* the agent that causes anthrax. An account of the recent history of this pathogen provides a window into the convergence of war, biomedicine, and financial speculation mobilized through the negative affects of fear, dread, and anxiety.

In Clinton's first year in office his administration established a market demand for products to contend with the presumed imminent threat of anthrax. In November 1993, under the direction of Clinton's first secretary of defense, Les Aspin, the Department of Defense issued Directive 6205.3, which established that military and civilian personnel assigned to "threat areas" and those designated for contingency deployment to these areas should be vaccinated against biological warfare threats. The initial assumption was that these threat areas were, for the most part, overseas. But provisions were also made for vaccinating researchers working stateside and for treating them with antidotes in the event of accidental or intentional exposure. General John Shalikashvili, Clinton's chairman of the Joint Chiefs of Staff, declared anthrax the primary biological warfare threat. Over the next few years the Department of Defense discussed how to implement the directive. On December 15, 1997, Secretary of Defense William S. Cohen announced preliminary plans to vaccinate all active and reserve armed forces members with a substance called Anthrax Vaccine Adsorbed (AVA). The goal was to offer maximum protection against the threat of weaponized anthrax.

Cohen's Total Force Anthrax Vaccine Immunization Program, or AVIP, was designed in three phases to be executed over a period of seven years. The program planned to use 15 million doses of vaccine to inoculate 2.4 million people, starting with personnel deployed to high-threat areas. During the first phase, all troops deployed to high-threat zones in Southwest Asia and the Korean Peninsula were to be vaccinated. Phase 2 was initially scheduled to begin in 2000 and would vaccinate "early deploying forces," active and reserve forces that were ordered to high-threat areas. Phase 3 was projected for 2003, when all remaining service members would be vaccinated regardless of their assigned duties. The immunization program consisted of a series of six inoculations for each service member over an eighteen-month period, followed by an annual booster. The plan was scheduled for implementation starting in May 1998. This, Cohen hoped, would give the Department of Defense sufficient time to make proper assessments for educating service members about the program, inspecting the production facilities, and confirming that the vaccine was safe and medically effective.

Almost immediately after AVIP was announced in 1993, service members across the military questioned the program. Many refused to be injected with the vaccine, citing Nuremburg conventions that require informed consent for medical experimentation. Their resistance was fueled by the military's neglectful treatment of Vietnam War–era veterans exposed to Agent Orange and of Persian Gulf War–era veterans who complained in vain of chronic fatigue, migraines, diarrhea, and nervous disorders related to Gulf War syndrome. The cause of the syndrome remained uncertain, but many who later refused to be inoculated under AVIP cited the not uncommon incidence of suffering among the estimated 150,000 U.S. troops vaccinated against anthrax prior to their deployment to the Persian Gulf in 1991.

At the time AVIP was established, only one facility in the United States was manufacturing vaccines against *Bacillus anthracis*, and it was hardly up to the task of producing the stockpile the program required. The story of how this facility went from a decrepit and substandard production plant to become part of a lucrative biotechnology start-up company in a little over a decade is peppered with elements of transnational intrigue, inside-the-beltway lobbying, dubious laboratory practices, slick corporate public relations campaigns, and the hubris that comes with being a sole-source contractor for a product that decision makers felt was urgently needed for the nation's survival and its future. The company's name, BioPort

Corporation, was a mash-up of the word *biology* and the place name *Porton Down*, home to the euphemistic Centre for Applied Microbiology and Research near Salisbury in Wiltshire, England, where clandestine weapons research had begun in 1916 in the aftermath of the German use of chemical warfare. In early 1998 BioPort, then a small start-up company with three principal investors, bid on an aging manufacturing plant and came away with what would become a key pretext for acquiring considerable amounts of government funding. It will be my case in point of a particular variant of war profiteering, one that sells biomedical products to parties at war.

PRIVATIZING BIOSECURITY

Located in the state capital of Lansing, the Michigan Biologic Products Institute (MBPI) was established in the early years of the twentieth century by the state's public health department. Its primary purpose was to develop vaccines. The institute received a license in 1970 from the National Institutes of Health to manufacture Anthrax Vaccine Adsorbed to prevent cutaneously transmitted anthrax. There are four different types of anthrax, classified by modes of transmission: inhalation (by breathing aerosolized spores), cutaneous (transmitted through cuts or scrapes on the skin after handling contaminated material), gastrointestinal (by eating raw or uncooked contaminated meat), and injection (by using contaminated needles). Human-to-human transmission is rare and is believed to occur when one person comes into contact with skin lesions of an infected person. The AVA manufactured by the facility in Lansing was for cutaneous anthrax only.

By the 1980s MBPI was the sole source manufacturer of the anthrax vaccine in the United States. Its customer base was small, mainly consisting of patients who handled infectious animal hides, the most common mode of transmission for cutaneous anthrax. In 1988 that customer base began to shift, as the U.S. Army signed a contract with the state of Michigan to increase the plant's output from 15,700 doses to 17,000 every four years to 300,000 in five years. But by the time the United States deployed troops to the Persian Gulf in 1991, the MBPI had produced only enough vaccine for 150,000 troops, a quarter of the amount needed to cover the projected 500,000.

The plant was in dire need of renovation, and Michigan decided to put it up for sale in 1996. Despite the Pentagon's offer to pay for a $1.8 million renovation, no buyers came forward. Circumstances changed dramatically in December 1997, when Secretary Cohen announced that all U.S. deployed troops and reservists would be vaccinated against anthrax in anticipation of going to war with Iraq in retaliation against Hussein's obstruction of UN weapons inspectors. Suddenly there was massive demand for AVA. Bids on the MBPI started coming in during January 1998, and by June the institute became the property of BioPort, which offered $24 million for it, $17 million to be paid up front and the rest in loans to be paid over the next five years. The sale offered the buyers an inside track on at least $60 million in Department of Defense contracts for anthrax vaccine.[28] It transferred the state-owned facility to a privately owned enterprise.

Meet the El-Hibri family, along with their well-connected co-investor. Fuad El-Hibri, a German businessman of Lebanese descent with a degree in economics from Stanford and another in public-private management from Yale University, was the principal investor and CEO of BioPort. His father, Ibrahim El-Hibri, a wealthy Venezuelan citizen who made a fortune in the telecommunications industry working for the Phillips Company in the Arab Gulf States, was a co-investor. The third investor was the former chairman of the Joint Chiefs of Staff under Reagan and George H. W. Bush, who served as Clinton's ambassador to the United Kingdom from 1994 to 1997, retired admiral William Crowe. Crowe and the elder El-Hibri met many years earlier through a mutual friend. Their paths crossed during the 1970s, when Crowe was head of the U.S. Central Command in Qatar. Ibrahim El-Hibri was in Qatar at the time, running several businesses. The men remained in contact during Crowe's years as ambassador. When Cohen announced the plan to conduct mass vaccinations of deployed U.S. troops in late 1997, Crowe, who had served on the board of the pharmaceutical giant Pfizer, strategized with the El-Hibris about taking over anthrax vaccine production in the United States since it had been so lucrative in the United Kingdom during the 1990s. Crowe encouraged Fuad El-Hibri to acquire his U.S. citizenship around the time of the purchase and was given 10 percent of BioPort's stock in return for his investment. Given Crowe's connections to the Pentagon, critics called it a rigged deal based on favoritism. He defended his actions by saying that the nation's defense against an anthrax attack was so urgent that if he could help answer the need he was justified in doing so.

During Operation Desert Storm, the Gulf War of 1990–91, Fuad El-Hibri had made a fortune working at a British company that sold anthrax vaccine. Taking advantage of Margaret Thatcher's privatization of previously state-owned industries in the 1980s, he and an acquaintance named Zsolt Harsanyi became involved in what was to become the world's largest biotechnology firm of its time, Porton International. Harsanyi was a U.S. citizen with a PhD in genetics, who was centrally involved in preparing an early report on biotechnology for the U.S. Office of Technology Assessment. As president of Porton International, Harsanyi and the younger El-Hibri succeeded in acquiring the rights to sell vaccines and other products produced by the Centre for Applied Microbiology and Research. The public funding of private enterprise that would come to dominate bioweapons research in the United States in the last years of the twentieth century started in England under Thatcher, and the El-Hibri family was there to take advantage.

Ibrahim El-Hibri became a silent partner in Porton International in 1989, as tensions in the Persian Gulf were growing and Hussein invaded Kuwait. Fuad was installed as director of a subsidiary called Porton Products. Father and son used their Middle East connections to sell tens of millions of dollars' worth of anthrax vaccine to Saudi Arabia and other countries in deals approved by the British Ministry of Defense. The price per dose for Saudis was $300 to $500, thirty to fifty times more than what the U.S. Department of Defense agreed to pay BioPort per dose nearly a decade later. In 1997 Porton International partnered with the huge defense contractor DynCorps, to form DynPort Vaccine Company. The new company was awarded a ten-year Department of Defense contract to the tune of $322 million to produce vaccines against various bacteria. So by the time BioPort bought MBPI, Fuad El-Hibri was already acquainted with the funding opportunities offered by the Pentagon.

BioPort got into trouble shortly after purchasing the Michigan facility. Substandard supplies of the AVA produced prior to the plant's renovation were delivered to military clinics and injected into troops who complained of headaches, joint pain, and memory loss. In addition the younger El-Hibri used government funds intended to upgrade the production facilities to remodel the executive offices in Michigan. Thousands of dollars were unaccounted for in an early round of auditing. Nevertheless, being a sole-source contractor, BioPort now had the leverage to demand more. Fuad testified before Congress in 1999 that his company would stop producing the anthrax vaccine if the Department of Defense did not agree to pay more for it: "Without a second market [a commercial market], the government cannot expect the rock-bottom pricing it enjoys with some of the other vaccines it purchases. . . . As a commercial entity, BioPort cannot continue to subsidize the Department of Defense."[29] The department complied by twice lowering the dose supply request and raising the price per dose, first from 8.7 million doses at $4.36 apiece to 7.9 million and then down to 4.6 million doses at $10.36 each. BioPort was also given an additional $24.1 million to facilitate production, roughly the entire purchase price the company had paid for the plant.

By 1999 the Department of Defense was on the hook for a lot of money and a large order of anthrax to fill. Despite earlier concerns about the Michigan plant's poor conditions, inspectors from the Food and Drug Administration visited the facility in September of that year and noted continuing progress. This allowed BioPort to submit a supplemental request for funds. But in October 2000 the FDA inspected the facility again and discovered faulty sterilizing procedures and found labels with inaccurate expiration dates on vials of the vaccine.[30] Despite this negative review, between 1998 and the end of 2001 the Pentagon gave BioPort almost $150 million, and yet by October 2001 the company had shipped no new vaccine.

The investigative journalist Laura Rozen found that large pharmaceutical companies are not inclined to bid for bioweapons contracts. Building and maintaining safe facilities is costly, and large companies prefer to produce a variety of drugs to serve larger numbers of patients. Part of the reason smaller, privately held corporations go after contracts for products like the anthrax vaccine is that they can count on being the sole-source contractor, which gives them a virtual monopoly on the product. Furthermore, unlike industry giants Merck, Pfizer, and GlaxoSmithKline, smaller start-ups generally do not have a commercial reputation to protect. Start-ups are privately held companies shielded from the scrutiny that publicly traded companies must deal with. I will return to BioPort since, despite its inefficiencies and graft, the company rebranded itself as more than just a single-product supplier and was given a big boost in the aftermath of the terrorist attacks of September and October 2001.

THE DOCTRINE OF PREEMPTION AND
POST-9/11 BIOSECURITY SURVEILLANCE

While Clinton was in his second term, the Project for a New American Century, a neoconservative think-tank based in Washington, D.C., began formulating a doctrine of preemption as part of its goal of expanding American global hegemony. The project was closely affiliated with the

American Enterprise Institute. Among its affiliates were Dick Cheney, the first President Bush's secretary of defense and the second Bush's vice president, and Donald Rumsfeld.[31] Among other initiatives, the project's doctrine of preemption urged the development of public-private partnerships aimed at enhancing the arsenal of biotechnological tools necessary to carry out military preemptive operations. In January 1998 a group of Republicans wrote a letter to Clinton requesting that he be willing to take military action against Iraq and to "turn your Administration's attention to implementing a strategy for removing Saddam's regime from power [since] diplomacy had failed."[32] Among the signatories were Elliott Abrams, assistant secretary of state for human rights and humanitarian affairs under Reagan; John Bolton, a staunch critic of the United Nations, whom George W. Bush appointed U.S. ambassador to the UN in 2005; Reagan's secretary of education, William J. Bennett; Paul Wolfowitz, a former assistant to the secretary of state under Reagan and undersecretary of defense for policy under George W. Bush; William Kristol, editor of the conservative *Weekly Standard*; and Rumsfeld, secretary of defense under Gerald Ford and George W. Bush. The group argued that Hussein was most likely developing weapons of mass destruction that he would use against Israel and America's Arab allies in the region. Such actions, they warned, would "put a significant portion of the world's supply of oil at hazard." Signatories to the letter would go on to be among the most outspoken proponents of George W. Bush's controversial doctrine of preemptive attack that was used to invade Iraq in March 2003.

Bush's administration combined what was called full-spectrum warfare with preemption to advance a future-oriented apparatus of military preparedness to handle real and imagined threats, including biological threats. Full-spectrum warfare is defined as a doctrine for gaining "full-spectrum superiority" through control over all dimensions of the "battlespace," including not only aerial, maritime, terrestrial, subterranean, and extraterrestrial spaces but also psychological, biological, and cybertechnological spaces.[33] Within the first year of his presidency Bush withdrew the United States from a United Nations effort to enforce the BTWC, a little over a month before the attacks of September 11, 2001. The terrorist operations that destroyed the World Trade Center and damaged the Pentagon were followed a few weeks later by news of deadly anthrax spores sent via the U.S. Postal Service. Together these events fueled fear and softened public criticism of preemptive attacks. Bush's U.S. National Security Strategy, announced on

September 20, 2002, allowed for preemptive actions and stressed the significance not just of *imminent* threats but also of *emergent* threats. Melinda Cooper explains that an emergent threat is one "whose actual occurrence remains irreducibly speculative, impossible to locate or predict."[34]

The doctrine of preemption and the idea of emergent threats rationalized new scientific research undertaken through DARPA funding, using the latest knowledge and techniques from recombinant DNA research and human genome mapping. In the name of biodefense, research to detect and protect against unknown threats authorized the creation of novel infectious pathogens and of more virulent strains of existing ones in order to engineer a cure. Researchers used a technique of DNA shuffling that was modeled on a scenario of anticipatory evolution.[35] They intentionally manufactured deadly strains in order to devise countermeasures for infectious diseases that did not yet exist. Since the research assumed an ongoing mutation or evolution of biological threats, the war against them was conceived as perpetual and permanent. When it came to biological weapons research, the boundary between wartime and peacetime was rendered a quaint illusion exceeding even that of the Cold War years, when the imminent threat of the nuclear bomb saturated public discourse and materialized in pedagogies of preparedness. With the coming of emergent threats—whose nature and capability were uncertain either because of rapid natural mutation or intentional gene splicing—the outdated doctrine of mutually assured destruction that kept the two superpowers in check gave way to speculation about what deadly agents could possibly be coming next. As early as 1998 this shift offered opportunities for established pharmaceutical companies as well as new biotechnology start-up companies to profit from a government mandate to develop and stockpile medical countermeasures in anticipation of intentional bioterrorist attacks and outbreaks of infectious diseases that were resistant to existing antibiotic and antiviral medicines.

In the wake of the attacks on 9/11 and the malicious anthrax mailings a month later, the Bush administration massively expanded the nation's security apparatus and developed a strategy to deal with biological attacks. The federal government would fund research to develop diagnostic tests and detection systems, to test and manufacturer effective vaccines, and to produce drugs to counter potential biological threats. One of the first initiatives of a newly created cabinet unit, the Department of Homeland Security, was Project BioWatch, a surveillance program designed to detect

pathogenic attacks and to gather forensic evidence for identifying perpetrators and for determining the scope of contamination.[36] In the first half
of 2003 the Environmental Protection Agency and the CDC worked together to roll out this massive system. With an initial budget of $533.8 mil-
lion, BioWatch activated detectors for airborne "bioterror agents" in thirty
cities across the United States. The system was labor-intensive and critics
questioned its efficacy: technicians were required to manually collect the
air filters and take them to laboratories for analysis, which created a delay
that undermined the early warning function of BioWatch. Among other
problems, regular air pollution caused false positives for biological contamination.[37]

Over the last months of 2002 the Department of Homeland Security
also established the U.S. National Biodefense Analysis and Countermeasures Center (NBACC) to study biological threats and develop defenses to
biological weapons attacks. Located at Fort Detrick, the NBACC included
the National Biodefense Analysis Center, conducting bioforensic analysis
of evidence from an attack by attaining a "biological fingerprint" of the
pathogen to assist in identifying perpetrators and to determine the origin
and method of the attack. It also included the National Biological Threat
Characterization Center, which was established to conduct laboratory experiments in order to understand current and future biological threats and
to evaluate vulnerabilities. This information was supposed to provide a
guide for developing countermeasures such as detection technologies, vaccines, pharmaceutical products, and decontamination systems. The Threat
Characterization Center was initially housed at the U.S. Army Medical Research Institute for Infectious Disease at Fort Detrick as a joint federal
effort bringing together the Department of Homeland Security, the FBI,
and the army. The Battelle National Biodefense Institute won the contract
to operate the NBACC and oversee the building of its laboratory within the
National Interagency Biodefense Campus at Fort Detrick. The government
owned the campus, and Battelle was given a contract to operate it.

From its inception, biosecurity experts concerned with arms control
and environmental safety criticized the NBACC.[38] Because it was designed
to develop and investigate genetically engineered pathogens, they argued
that the NBACC could be in violation of the BTWC rule against developing and stockpiling biological weapons.[39] The NBACC was also equipped
with biocontainment facilities in which to conduct tests of deadly pathogens on laboratory animals and, if necessary, to quarantine people who

were infected with lethal viruses. Classified as a Sensitive Compartmented Information Facility, the Biological Threat Characterization Center was, critics believed, cordoned off from public scrutiny in the name of security and exempted from the usual system of peer-reviewed science and ethics review. The Department of Homeland Security was charged with making sure the Center was operating in compliance with arms control treaties, but this amounted to an internal review because the reviewers were senior DHS officials who were involved in the research themselves.[40] Critics also questioned whether there were sufficient safeguards against the growing number of staff members at the Center who might be in the position to leak classified data or use biological materials to harm others. Furthermore they noted that the Center, which was to include laboratories equipped to deal with the most dangerous pathogens known to humans, could endanger local populations.[41] Another common criticism was that the synthetic DNA resulting from genetic engineering produced at the NBACC and at privately contracted commercial laboratories was not sufficiently regulated and could easily fall into the hands of biohackers who could use it to launch attacks.[42] The Bush administration responded by claiming it was in compliance with the BTWC because its programs were strictly defensive. Manufacturing small amounts of pathogens, they argued, was necessary for research. It also concluded that the NBACC facility would pose no environmental risks and its staff would be carefully monitored to prevent the misuse of data and research materials.[43]

Congress approved legislation authorizing Project BioShield in July 2004, placing the Department of Health and Human Services and the Department of Homeland Security jointly in charge of the program. Project BioShield was part of the effort to develop vaccines and drugs and received initial funding in 2004 of $5.6 billion to grant to commercial and academic laboratories with promising products in the pipeline. The legislation relaxed procedures for some CBRN terrorism-related spending, such as research grants and hiring, and it permitted emergency use of unapproved measures.[44] It expedited the normal peer review process, awarding grants within three to five months of the application deadline instead of the usual nine to eighteen. Under this new plan the federal government authorized $5.593 billion for ten years to purchase vaccines in the amount of $2.3 billion, with the remainder to be spent on research to produce a variety of countermeasures against what were assumed to be imminent or emergent biological attacks.

Project BioShield money was restricted to developing drugs for which there was no commercial market. This guaranteed researchers and pharmaceutical companies that the federal government would pay for what they developed in countermeasures to rare outbreaks. The legislation stipulated that funds could not be used to procure countermeasures or treat harm resulting from any "naturally occurring infectious disease or other public health threat." Funds were restricted to medical countermeasures against intentional biological attacks. Congress assumed that anthrax exposure, while highly disruptive, was likely to affect a much smaller number of people. Big pharmaceutical companies did not want to invest in developing products with such a small market. But small start-ups were happy to receive the funds, as were scientists working in government laboratories seeking support for basic research. Their principal customer would be the U.S. government. Project BioShield's distinction between "natural" and "intentional" outbreaks was in practice vague and questionable. But the funding restrictions served as a firewall against legislative raids that would take money earmarked for homeland security and either give it to big corporations rather than government researchers or use it to restore primary public health care that had been slashed by a Republican-controlled Congress.

The National Institutes of Health, part of the Department of Health and Human Services (HHS), received funding for basic research through BioShield. Its National Institute of Allergy and Infectious Diseases, based in Bethesda, Maryland, got $1.5 billion in 2003 and by 2011 had received $14 billion for biodefense research. The tempo accelerated in 2006, when BARDA was created within the Office of the Assistant Secretary for Preparedness and Response in the HHS. Its mission was to take new concepts and products into further development and testing. Eventually BARDA was assigned to oversee Project BioShield.

BARDA provided funds to encourage academic and commercial laboratories to move products from the laboratory to the market by covering their costs across the "Valley of Death," the long period consumed by clinical trials to determine a drug's efficacy and safety. Many commercially developed drugs did not make it past this valley, either because they failed in clinical trials or the market for them was too small to be profitable. BARDA offered a bridge across the valley. As one researcher remarked, "You can think of BARDA almost like a venture capital firm buried in the U.S. Government."[45] An added benefit to the researchers was that, unlike venture capitalists, the government would not expect a portion of the profits.

BARDA was funded under legislation originally introduced by Senator Richard Burr, who sponsored the Biodefense and Pandemic Vaccine and Drug Development Act of 2005 (S1873) just two weeks after the debate over the Harkin amendment to the Defense Appropriations bill concerning avian influenza. Burr's proposed bill exempted pharmaceutical companies from any liability for death or injury caused by their drug or vaccine if it was designated as a countermeasure. It also shielded participating pharmaceutical companies from public scrutiny in order to protect their proprietary interests. The Pharmaceutical Research and Manufacturers of America lobbied for the legislation. Burr argued that it was an improvement on Project BioShield because it guaranteed confidentiality, which would attract more companies.[46] The exemption from open records laws that applied to most government departments would, he claimed, "provide the incentives and protections necessary to bring more and better drugs and vaccines to market faster."[47] Burr received $288,684 from drug companies during his first year in the Senate, making him the top recipient of pharmaceutical campaign money that year.[48] The bill went down to defeat in Congress after critics warned that its confidentiality and no-liability clauses were in violation of patients' rights. But Burr and his supporters regrouped to design a slightly modified bill.

A little over a year later, on December 5, 2006, a press release from Burr's office announced that the Senate had approved Senate Bill 3678, "Pandemic and All-Hazards Preparedness Act," a revised version of S1873. Burr's press release read, "The Biomedical Advanced Research and Development Authority (BARDA) *will be an aggressive venture capitalist partnering with universities, research institutions and industry on the advanced development of promising drugs and vaccines*. . . . The bill improves our ability to quickly develop countermeasures to protect against deadly threats such as pandemic flu and bioterrorism. The process for developing a new drug or vaccine still takes up to a decade and costs hundreds of millions of dollars."[49] The revised version removed the exemption that would have allowed a no-liability status for drug companies. It did, however, maintain a guarantee of confidentiality "in accordance with the exception from the public discourse of trade secrets" (Section 319.Ac) and a limited antitrust exemption to facilitate communication among parties to the development of medical countermeasures.[50] Because BARDA was set up to expedite research and development of countermeasures, it allowed for sole-source contracts. The legislation passed by unanimous consent in both the Senate and House and was signed by Bush on December 19, 2006.

The Department of Defense meanwhile had its own semi-autonomous program to deal with biological attacks. In 2006 it established the Transformational Medical Technologies (TMT) initiative. Originally conceived as a five-year project and budgeted at $1.5 billion, the program aimed at accelerating the development of countermeasures to protect soldiers against biological attacks. It became permanent in 2009. Its goals were to sequence the genomes of potential bioterror agents, explore new drug technologies, and develop broad-spectrum therapies that would work against multiple bacterial and viral pathogens. Some TMT projects were eventually folded into other Pentagon efforts, and by 2011 TMT became part of the Defense Threat Reduction Agency. Critics complained that the initiative was a waste of money because the only drug that made it into a clinical trial is one for fighting influenza, a disease that was already heavily researched in civilian and commercial laboratories.[51] Like so many other efforts for developing and manufacturing effective vaccines and drugs to counter biological pathogens, TMT failed to deliver faster and more effective antibiotic therapies. Its defenders argued that five years was not enough time to move a therapy from basic research through approval and mass manufacturing. TMT provided contracts to small start-up companies who were willing to take on more risk than big companies. But many of these small contractors also lacked experience and certain necessary skills for moving a product toward manufacturing and scaling up for mass stockpiling.

By the end of 2006 Congress had allocated a new round of billions of dollars for research on medical countermeasures. This was welcome news to those in the drug industry. When pharmaceutical company representatives say that it costs between $800 million and $1 billion to develop, test, gain approval, and market a single drug, that represents a substantial amount of taxpayers' money. Many of the larger pharmaceutical companies showed little interest in making such an investment when the market for products was so esoteric. Their attitude shifted when the government promised to buy up what they produced. Biodefense funding was a considerable stimulus package for biotechnology companies.[52] Rising stock prices reflected this.

By the turn of the twenty-first century, biotechnology companies were following in the footsteps of conventional weapons manufacturers and defense strategy management firms who had for decades been benefiting from long-term government contracts. As we have seen in the case of BioPort and its subsidiaries, government contracts offered the advantages of long-term support and a virtual monopoly as a sole-source supplier.

Public-private partnerships channeled taxpayers' money into private enterprises, which were able to exploit worries about war and terrorism. With the passage of the Patent and Trademark Law Amendments (the Bayh-Dole Act of 1980), inventions made with federal funding no longer belonged to the government but could instead be owned by the company, university, or nonprofit organization responsible for the invention. This meant that the contracting businesses or universities were permitted to exclusively license the inventions to other parties (i.e., collect funds for licensing the invention). The opportunities afforded by Bayh-Dole to biotechnology companies were vast.[53] War, terrorism, and the fear of disease outbreaks provided the conditions for scaling up production of countermeasures, stimulating the political will for Congress and the executive branch to approve vast expenditures on government contracts given to private laboratories, even in the midst of evidence of modest practical returns, a great amount of inefficiency, and no small measure of extortion by contractors.

"TO PROTECT AND ENHANCE"

Let us return for a moment to the BioPort Corporation since its history offers an illuminating example of how imminent and emergent threats provide lucrative and speculative economic opportunities through biomedical war profiteering. After temporarily losing its license to produce anthrax vaccine in 2001, BioPort's license was restored in early 2002 partly due to panic stemming from the malicious anthrax mailings. In 2002 the company increased its spending on lobbyists from $30,000 to $110,000 and then to $220,000 in 2003. A year to the day after the attacks of 9/11 an expert panel of doctors, scientists, and former military officers recommended that the government purchase more of BioPort's product. The company paid several members of the panel to review and endorse the report, which was ghost-written by the staff of BioPort. In September 2003, when the Pentagon was paying $22 a dose, more than double the price negotiated in the 1999 bailout, BioPort became a subsidiary of Emergent BioSolutions. El-Hibri and his business partners headed up the new venture. At the end of 2003 Emergent BioSolutions announced that it had purchased a Maryland drug maker for more than $3 million and signed a contract with the Pentagon worth between $29.7 million and $245 million, depending on the number of doses sold. In 2004 the rebranded company began building a second $95 million anthrax vaccination plant in Frederick, Maryland. Fuad

El-Hibri never moved to Michigan to oversee the old plant but remained in the Washington, D.C., area, where he was planning to build a commercial equestrian and polo center near the family's home in Gaithersburg, Maryland, roughly equidistant from BioPort's corporate offices in Washington and Frederick. The state of Maryland gave Emergent BioSolutions funds in exchange for creating local jobs.

In January 2005 the company signed a deal with the British government to work cooperatively on developing toxoid and botulism vaccines. Several weeks later Emergent purchased a British company working on five vaccines, including an oral anthrax vaccine. Following Project BioShield's passage, the company was awarded a five-year contract for 2004–9 in the amount of $690 million to produce 29 million doses of the FDA-approved anthrax vaccine named BioThrax. In 2011 it won another five-year contract to provide 44.8 million doses of BioThrax to the Strategic National Stockpile in a deal worth up to $1.25 billion. In 2013 the company acquired the exclusive right to manufacture and sell VaxInnate, an anti-influenza vaccine composed of recombinant DNA. Emergent BioSolutions purchased the Canadian biotech company Cangene in February 2014, which brought three other specialty products into the company's portfolio designed to counter botulism and inhalation anthrax. In 2015 the company got another $31 million from BARDA/HHS to develop an improved version called Nu-Thrax. Based on FDA approval for Anthrasil in 2015, an injected medicine for treating people with anthrax, the company received $7 million from BARDA. The company's revenue in 2015 was $540 million, up from $100 million the previous year.

BioPort's corporate makeover was signified by a name that combined a grammar of anticipation (Emergent) with aspiration (Solutions), held together by the signifier of life (Bio). Attached to its mashed-up name was a new slogan, "To Protect and Enhance," a promissory gesture marking the distance from running a substandard vaccine plant out in the Midwest to aspiring to become a twenty-first-century cutting-edge biotechnology innovator whose products promised to do more than prepare us for doomsday. "One Emergent Culture," a cloying promotional video on the company's website, emphasizes the firm's corporate culture of "speaking in a united voice" and "working as a team toward one goal: to save lives" as the camera zooms in on a vial of BioThrax. The company's publicity emphasizes products that are not apparently tied to biodefense, including drugs for hemophilia B, leukemia, and prostate cancer. Its public relations campaign stresses how much the company cares about health. Emergent BioSolutions had indeed appeared to overcome its sordid reputation when it was announced in 2012 as one of three public-private partnerships named by Obama as a BARDA Center for Innovation in Advanced Development and Manufacturing. The award came with an eight-year $220 million contract to develop medical countermeasures to a variety of threats.

Between 2001 and 2011 the federal government paid out $19 billion on biodefense research across all of its agencies and institutions, out of a full allocation for biosecurity of $60 billion.[54] The cost far exceeded the benefit to the public. In 2010 the bipartisan, congressionally mandated Commission on the Prevention of Mass Destruction Proliferation and Terrorism gave the federal government an "F" for its efforts to "enhance the nation's capabilities for rapid response to prevent biological attacks from inflicting mass casualties."[55] Also in 2010 a body of experts that guided the HHS concerning its biodefense projects concluded that the nation lacked a unified strategy that would focus on the leading threats and develop the best responses. The American public, it noted, "expects orchestration within HHS's scientific endeavors, not cacophony" when it comes to responding to biological threats.[56]

In an attempt to deal with the noted inefficiencies, in June 2012 the Obama administration established the Centers for Innovation in Advanced Development and Manufacturing, the body that had awarded Emergent BioSolutions its $220 million contract. Obama lifted the funding restrictions of Project BioShield by allowing this new domestic infrastructure to generate drugs for biological defense as well as for other public health purposes. The centers were to be administered by HHS through BARDA. The plan set up three teams, consisting of public-private partnerships of for-profit companies, government research centers, and research universities. Initial funding amounted to around $400 million. Promoted as a more efficient way to conduct research, the program would build new facilities for developing cell-based and recombinant-based vaccines for dealing with pandemic influenza and other imminent and emergent threats. Private companies would provide about a third of the funding in the initial building phase, while the HHS, using taxpayers' money, would provide the other two-thirds and would pay for the operation and maintenance of the Centers for the subsequent years. The move also allowed contracts to be renewed for up to twenty-five years, signaling a long-term commitment to the partnership between the federal government and industry.

Establishing the Centers for Innovation was a response to a Public Health Emergency Medical Review requested by the secretary of HHS, Kathleen Sebelius, after her department encountered substantial congressional obstacles for developing countermeasures, especially during the H1N1 pandemic flu wave in 2009 that infected an estimated 1 million people in the United States. The United States reported the greatest number of H1N1 cases worldwide, but most of the ill recovered without requiring medical treatment.[57] Nevertheless Sebelius was concerned that the nation had not been adequately prepared for such a pandemic. So the Centers for Innovation were essentially set up as manufacturing plants to help small companies produce commercial quantities of drugs and vaccines. Despite the original hope that HHS would work with the Department of Defense to build the facilities together, the two agencies set up separate operations. Once again the Department of Defense asserted that its priority was protecting troops with vaccines against potential bioweapons, while the National Institute of Allergy and Infectious Diseases, part of HHS, prioritized fundamental microbial sequencing and vaccine development for all kinds of biothreats, whether introduced in terrorist attacks or by natural causes. The articulated goal of establishing a coordinated domestic infrastructure that would cut costs, avoid duplication, and be more effective in protecting the nation against biological attacks was once again undermined by differing institutional interests. News of the costliness and inefficiency of the nation's biodefense infrastructure contributed to the public's wariness and mistrust already aroused by revelations about how injured troops and veterans were inadequately treated at Walter Reed Army Medical Center and other Veterans Administration facilities around the country.[58]

BIOSECURITY AND DISPOSABLE LIFE

Public suspicion over military-related research on pathogens and uses of experimental countermeasures had a long but mostly forgotten history before the anthrax scare of 2001. A Senate report from 1994 asserted that the public has been intentionally exposed to potentially dangerous substances without their knowledge or consent, covering events going back to the research initiated in the 1940s at Fort Detrick.[59] It reviewed a long history of experiments that used military personnel as research subjects, cautioning that even in cases where participation was voluntary, subjects were not always sufficiently informed of the dangers. The report discussed the history of veterans' radiation exposure from 1945 to 1962, primarily in the South Pacific. It also criticized experiments conducted by the CIA using LSD and other hallucinogens, including quinuclidinyl benzilate ("BZ" or "Buzz"), which were weaponized to serve as incapacitating agents. The report, issued by the Senate Committee on Veterans Affairs, recounted that from 1943 to 1973 the U.S. biological weapons program staged more than two hundred domestic tests aimed at assessing the national vulnerability to biological warfare. These included nine months of testing bombs containing botulism on Horn Island, off the Mississippi coast, in 1943. In 1953 the U.S. Army Chemical Corps created the St. Jo Program, which staged mock anthrax attacks in St. Louis, Minneapolis, and Winnipeg, releasing bacteria that simulated anthrax from generators mounted on cars. During 1950 researchers at Fort Detrick developed the yellow fever virus in order to infect enemies by releasing mosquitoes from airplanes and helicopters. In 1965 the army's Special Operations Division spread bacteria throughout Washington's National Airport. The following year the division dropped lightbulbs filled with organisms onto New York City subway tracks from fast-moving trains to see how far the germs would be dispersed. In 1950 the U.S. Army clandestinely sprayed the bacterium *Serratia marcescens* across the city of San Francisco to see how fast and far the bacteria would travel. A seventy-five-year-old pipe fitter, Edward J. Nevins, came down with a fever and was admitted to a local hospital, where he died three weeks later from *Serratia* infection.[60] Similar secret experiments were conducted in Florida, Minnesota, and New York City during these decades.

Harriet Washington, an award-winning medical writer, has recently unearthed the sordid history of the U.S. government's targeting of African American communities for secret biological weapons testing.[61] Following World War II, under Jim Crow racial segregation, African Americans were concentrated in dilapidated housing infested with vermin and "glazed with lead paint." Health care for people in these communities was nonexistent. In the summer of 1951 the state of Florida built a 466-unit addition to a large apartment complex in Miami originally opened in 1946. Named after George Washington Carver, the addition was finally opened to black people in a new town called Carver Village. It was the largest and most impressive new housing development for black people in the nation. Shortly after it opened the Ku Klux Klan descended on Miami riding motorcycles and terrorizing the community. Between September and the end of the year they bombed an empty building in the complex and several Jewish schools and synagogues around Miami, exploded dynamite in Carver Village, and bombed a Catholic church that was associated with the antisegregationist movement. In December 1951 terrorists destroyed two more Jewish synagogues to punish Jewish supporters of desegregation, and on Christmas the leader of the Florida NAACP was assassinated in a bombing.

Throughout most of the 1950s, Washington writes, "another silent species of violence, this time at the hands of the U.S. government," was under way amid the overt vigilante violence being carried out by segregationists.[62] The U.S. Army Special Operations Division at Fort Detrick produced chemical and biological weapons with first-strike capability. Since 1952 it had partnered with the Central Intelligence Agency in a program code-named MK-NAOMI. As part of MK-NAOMI the U.S. Army Chemical Corps bred more than 4 million mosquitoes a day at Fort Detrick. The mosquitoes were released in swarms near Carver Village to determine if they could function as disease vectors and, if so, whether they could be used as first-strike biological weapons to spread infectious diseases such as yellow fever and malaria. In 1955 the government targeted another black neighborhood in Florida. Because it bordered a white neighborhood, both groups were infected with whooping cough virus that led to a dozen deaths. That same year residents of Palmetto, on Florida's west coast, experienced a spike in cases of whooping cough. Carver Village sustained the greatest toll: over a thousand people came down with the disease. By 1960 Carver Village's residents were plagued with other mysterious diseases, including symptoms of dengue and yellow fever, some resulting in death.

Under the clandestine MK-NAOMI and MK-ULTRA programs, residents of another Carver Village, in Georgia, not far from Savannah, were sickened by an experiment involving mosquitoes undertaken in 1955 and 1956.[63] Residents recall young white men coming by their homes to inform them they were setting traps to see how far mosquitoes would travel, mentioning nothing else. The boxes were filled with mosquitoes that swarmed and infected residents, leading to illness and death in some cases. In 1973 Sidney Gottlieb, the program's director, destroyed the paper trail of the years of secret experimentation. Patient advocates and local citizens of Carver Village, Georgia, organized and filed a Freedom of Information Act request for materials related to MK-ULTRA's activities. The few documents that they received were enough to indicate regular train travel between CIA headquarters and Carver Village, Florida. Among them were receipts for the purchase of test animals, chemicals, and the hiring of a crop duster. There were also receipts for *Hemophilus pertussis* dated 1955, the year of the whooping cough outbreak. The evidence uncovered through the FOIA request revealed that at least until 1972 the U.S. government was waging a war of domestic terrorism against some of its most vulnerable citizens.[64]

In relatively recent history the plight of Persian Gulf War veterans serves as another troubling case of government malfeasance. The 1994 Senate report cited the exposure of U.S. troops in the Persian Gulf War to investigational drugs, including pyridostigmine bromide, a nerve agent that was believed to offer a form of protection from nerve gas attacks. According to the Department of Defense, all 696,562 U.S. troops in the Persian Gulf War were issued pyridostigmine bromide as a pretreatment for nerve agent poisoning. The department claimed that these doses were administered on a voluntary basis, but a substantial majority whom the Senate committee interviewed (74 percent of the seventy-three individuals interviewed who were given the bromide) said they were offered no choice.[65] About eight thousand individuals received botulinum toxoid and also reported lack of informed and uncoerced consent. The committee noted that the safety of these substances had not been verified, nor had the vaccine against the anthrax bacterium. It concluded that the Department of Defense and the Department of Veterans Affairs "repeatedly failed to provide information and medical follow-up to those who participate in military research or are ordered to take investigational drugs."[66] War is an occasion for medical experimentation, and the bodies of lower ranking service men and women, like those of African American residents of the Carver Villages of Florida and Georgia, are especially disadvantaged and threatened by these violent practices.

Another sordid chapter in domestic terrorism originating from within the U.S. government manifested in the very different official responses to the anthrax-laced letters mailed a few weeks after 9/11. Congressional offices that received envelopes were immediately evacuated, sealed, and decontaminated and their staff members tested for exposure to anthrax spores. By contrast, the U.S. Brentwood Mail Processing and Distribution Center in Washington, D.C., where 92 percent of the 2,646 employees were African American, remained open even after it became known that the contaminated envelopes had been sent through machines and handled by workers. The U.S. Postal Service did not address the issue until three days later, offering the affected workers a sixty-day antibiotic treatment but failing to mention that the treatment might not be sufficient to protect them. The workers were also told they were eligible for an experimental anthrax vaccine but would need to accept responsibility for any side effects from the treatment. The delayed intervention and the mixed messages they received about risks and possible benefits raised workers' suspicions. Why were they being told about the need for various treatments, some of which were risky, when they were initially told their workplace was not dangerous and they were at low risk for infection? Some, justifiably, believed that they were being offered the vaccine as part of an undisclosed experiment rather than as a treatment. Postal workers at the Morgan Station Center in New York City protested that they were being treated differently from the congressional staff members and, through their union, demanded the facility be closed and decontaminated before they would come back to work. The Postal Service refused to close the facility or test the employees. Instead it gave them a ten-day supply of the antibiotic drug Cipro, latex gloves, and paper masks. A third of the workers joined a boycott, but to little avail. The Postal Service decontaminated the processing machines but not the building. Willie Smith, the New York Metro Postal Union's president, told a *New York Times* reporter, "I realize that Morgan employees are not Supreme Court justices or senators or congressmen, but they are God's children. . . . They have the same right to life as the aristocrats. No one piece of mail is worth a human life."[67] As a result of the delayed intervention, four postal workers came down with inhalation anthrax, and two of them died.

The history of biological weapons research in the United States is marked by episodes of government officials endangering the lives of ordinary people, whether by releasing infected mosquitoes in African American neighborhoods or neglecting to take care of postal workers exposed to anthrax spores or by subjecting lower-ranking military personnel to dangerous biological agents in covert experiments and in risky vaccination campaigns. These episodes belie the social contract, according to which a democratic government is supposed to protect the citizens it represents. Post-9/11 public anxiety about biological threats stems in part from some communities' awareness of this blighted history. Though the post-9/11 counterterror state emphasized the threats posed by the infected migrant and the foreign terrorist with WMD, public revelations that the greatest perpetrators of biological threats to the United States in recent years were government officials added to the malaise that attached ordinary people to war through a state of disgusted suspicion. In a strange twist of fate, on July 29, 2008, Bruce Ivins, a top biodefense research scientist at the U.S. Army's headquarters for research and development of defensive biological weapons, committed suicide by overdosing on Tylenol. Ivins, who worked at the facility at Fort Detrick for eighteen years, was a prime suspect in the anthrax attacks. About a week after his death, the Department of Justice announced that he was solely responsible for the deaths and injuries, basing their finding on evidence they collected during a raid of his home while he was hospitalized for depression. There is considerable doubt among some of his coworkers and others familiar with the case about whether he was the perpetrator. But the very idea that a career biodefense researcher was the main suspect in a highly disruptive domestic terrorist attack amplified the public perception that the nation was vulnerable from within.

ENTER GILEAD

The H5N1 influenza pandemic that Senator Harkin and others predicted in 2005 did not come to pass in the United States. Though some cases of infected poultry were reported, the CDC announced in January 2015 that no cases of human infection had been detected in the United States.[68] But there is an interesting twist to this story. As the senators were arguing in late 2005 about restoring funds to the NIH and CDC through an addition to the 2006 Defense Appropriations bill, a California biotechnology company was poised to make a fortune on government orders for its leading product. Gilead Sciences, named after the Old Testament passages about the miraculously healing balm from the mountainous region of Gilead (now part of modern-day Jordan), held the rights to Tamiflu, an anti-influenza remedy touted as the most sought-after drug in the world in the wake of the panic over avian flu's imminent arrival in the United States.[69] Gilead Sciences was established in Brisbane, California, in 1987, one of the many new biotechnology companies springing up along the corridor just south of San Francisco, a short driving distance from Stanford University, UC Berkeley, UC San Francisco Medical Center, and the booming technology region of Silicon Valley. In July 2005 the Pentagon ordered $58 million worth of Tamiflu for U.S. troops around the world while Congress was considering a multibillion dollar purchase to prepare for an H5N1 outbreak. The drug, which does not cure the flu but can lessen the severity of symptoms if taken soon enough after infection, is manufactured and marketed by the

Swiss-based Roche Pharmaceutical. Gilead Sciences receives a royalty from Roche of about 10 percent of sales. Roche anticipated sales for Tamiflu during 2005 to be about $1 billion, up from $258 million in 2004.

By the time the congressional hearings of 2005 rolled around, Gilead Sciences enjoyed the reputation of being the most politically well-connected biotechnology company in the United States. Rumsfeld had served on the board of directors from 1988 to 2001 and was its chairman from 1997 until he joined the Bush administration as secretary of defense in 2001. Though he then recused himself from any decisions involving Gilead, he retained his stock holdings. Stock in Gilead traded between $6.64 and $17.93 in 2001. By 2005 Rumsfeld's stock was valued at between $5 million and $25 million, according to federal financial disclosures he was required to file. Between April and October 2005, during the growing panic over H5N1, Gilead's stock climbed from $35 to $47 a share. Between January and April 2006 its price range was $53 to $65.62. George Schultz, former secretary of state under Reagan, another member of Gilead's board of directors, sold more than $7 million worth of stock in the company between January and October 2005. Rumsfeld, already one of the wealthiest members of the Bush cabinet, had earned at least $1 million when Gilead's stock increased in value during the latter half of 2005. And the United States was only one of more than sixty countries that ordered Tamiflu to add to their national stockpiles.

Harkin and his colleagues in the Senate who argued for restoring funding for the CDC and the NIH were probably less concerned with lining the pockets of Tamiflu shareholders and more with keeping their Republican opponents from gutting the nation's public health infrastructure. They chose to cast their argument in a rhetoric of war against a foreign menace, hoping that panic over avian flu and its threat to national security would make it politically unwise for Republication Congress members to go along with the Bush administration's proposed cuts to the nation's public health infrastructure. Harkin and the Democrats did not prevail. Under a Republican-controlled Congress in 2011–13 annual funding for the CDC's Public Health Emergency Preparedness and Response Capability declined from a high of $1.09 billion in 2006 to $585 million in 2013, a 50 percent cut. For 2013 the program's budget was $1 billion lower than it had been in 2002, the first funding year after the attacks of 9/11 and the anthrax attacks. Between 2008 and 2013 the CDC lost 45,700 jobs at state and local health departments, hampering emergency preparedness and response efforts.

Harkin and his Senate colleagues' efforts to evade the budget cuts targeted by Republicans against the nation's leading centers of public health research and treatment were only partially successful. In 2006 Senator Harkin's amendment to the $107 billion Emergency Supplemental Appropriations bill was passed by the Senate on April 4. The amendment allocated $2.3 billion to prepare for an influenza epidemic, while $67.8 billion was to go to the Pentagon to support the war in Iraq and $27 billion was earmarked for hurricane relief.[70] The CDC and the NIH temporarily staved off the worst of the budget cuts that they would eventually suffer, especially after the Great Recession that began in December 2007.

Though the predicted epidemic of H5N1 did not strike the United States, the prospect of future outbreaks of virulent epidemics had been mobilized as a way to make up for serious losses in funding for public health research, clear evidence of the desperate conditions caused by privatizing biosecurity and forgoing meaningful and effective public health provision.

SYNOPSIS

Manufacturers of medical countermeasures exploited the anxiety that followed the anthrax attacks of 2001 and the fear that Colin Powell unleashed when he asserted before the UN that it was time to wage a preemptive war against the regime of Saddam Hussein. The fear of imminent and emergent biological threats helped pharmaceutical companies such as Emergent BioSolutions and Gilead Sciences to lobby for and acquire government contracts. Through vast expenditures propelled by fear of impending threats, logics of war have become further embedded in the development of medical knowledge of our time. Biomedical scientists have done more than respond to the wounds caused by war; some also concocted dangerous pathogens in order to engineer countermeasures. Over the past three decades a structured silence about industry-generated risks abetted the entanglements of public health, microbiology, and genetic engineering with a doctrine of preemptive and ongoing war. One outcome of this silence is that lower ranking military personnel, economically disadvantaged communities of color, and animals used in research became particularly subject to injury in experiments that exposed them to sickening and deadly pathogens. The hoped-for security for the privileged was staged through the intentionally inflicted risks to the disempowered, often against their knowledge and certainly without their consent.

While conducting the early research for this book, from the first years of the wars in Afghanistan and Iraq, I was struck by how little was published in the leading American medical journals about the illness and injury experiences of ordinary Afghan and Iraqi people, those whom our government ostensibly liberated through regime change. What I did notice in my survey of the *Journal of the American Medical Association* and the *New England Journal of Medicine* is that the few articles that discussed the health of Afghans and Iraqis were about infectious diseases. I discovered a disturbing pattern of concern about the spread of antibiotic-resistant tuberculosis and other respiratory diseases whose increasing virulence was being partially attributed to "noncompliant patients"—patients who do not take the full course of antibiotics prescribed to them and therefore whose actions contribute to the mutation of the pathogen in question.

Violent conflict, especially on the scale carried out in those two theaters of war, disrupted lives, unleashed mass migrations, destroyed health clinics and hospitals, killed doctors and nurses, and radically diminished many individuals' experience of health, compromising the immune system and contributing to malnutrition and intense psychological and physical stress. Massive aerial bombing and stockpiling arsenals of munitions degraded the air quality, exacerbating respiratory diseases. I found very little discussion of these issues and almost nothing about the traumatic brain injuries, limb loss, and posttraumatic stress among the occupied peoples in my survey of the literature. Instead it seemed that the main and possibly only concern for these people in our medical journals was that they may be responsible for the rise of ever more virulent strains of bacteria and viruses that have the potential to spread far, wide, and fast. The unequal economy of life I have been preoccupied with in this book manifests in how infectious disease agents are regarded as enemy agents in times of war and who, moreover, is seen to be at risk for infection by them.

Through the regime of global health security the U.S. counterterrorist state's concern for biosecurity went planetary. Preparing for imminent and emergent threats was part of a broadly conceived strategy of preemption in which conflict and danger are staged as ongoing. To the extent that research on biological threats claims to advance scientific knowledge, biosecurity functions as a rationale in the mutual provocation between war and biomedicine that I have referred to as biomedical salvationism. Postpolytrauma rehabilitative therapeutics and bionic prosthetics research, however problematic, aim to restore hope to patients and to a witnessing public by demonstrating novel devices and products. They have a palliative dimension. By contrast, biodefense research raises the specter of imminent and future risks that threaten potentially everyone. It medicalizes the nation in the allegorical sense of protecting it from foreign pathogens. It performs much of its work in secret. It invests in technological solutions to microscopic matters rather than considering the larger political factors that cause bio-insecurity in the first place. Chief among them are imperialist invasions, environmental destruction, forced migration, and ongoing war.

Epilogue

I opened this book with a story about praying for my father's future in the wake of his surviving severe war-generated injuries. The wars he fought damaged his body and his spirit and led him to die an early and painful death on a gurney in the hallway of a Veterans Hospital. His suffering had a profound effect on the people he loved and who loved him. Our family's story is not unique. Millions have gone through the pain of dying in the name of national belonging. Even more have perished in the brutal violence wrought by modern imperial wars fought in the name of humanity.

How do we loosen the attachments that tie us to war? How can we imagine and practice different ways of world-making that sunder

Learning to stay with the trouble of living and dying together on a damaged earth will prove more conducive to the kind of thinking that would provide the means to building more livable futures. . . . Our task is to make trouble, to stir up potent response to devastating events, as well as to settle troubled waters and rebuild quiet places. In urgent times, many of us are tempted to address trouble in terms of making an imagined future safe, of stopping something from happening that looms in the future, of clearing away the present and the past in order to make futures for coming generations. Staying with the trouble does not require such a relationship to times called the future. In fact, staying with the trouble requires learning to be truly present, not as a vanishing pivot between awful or edenic pasts and apocalyptic or salvific futures, but as mortal critters entwined in myriad unfinished configurations of places, times, matters, meanings.

—DONNA J. HARAWAY, *Staying with the Trouble*

the relationship between deliberate violence and the technosalvific logic of the biomedicine-war nexus? I have argued for intervening in the biomedical logics that tie medicine to war, first, by identifying where, when, and how they operate. Biomedical logics that associate medicine with an ethic of care have functioned to obscure the root causes and effects of violence in war. Discourses of care and benevolence have been used to authorize harmful security measures and to rationalize, retrospectively, the profound damage caused by war. Biomedical logics are evident in the common narrative that credits war and violence with the capability of advancing knowledge and therefore serving an abstraction called "humanity." Undoing this common narrative is part of the work of world-making that stays with the trouble by living and practicing peaceful modes of care. We can think of world-making also in terms of what Katie Stewart has theorized in her use of *worlding*. She uses the word to trace communities of copresence and coexperience that form around conditions, practices, pleasures, scenes of absorption, forms of attunement and attachment, and often fleeting strategies for self-transformation. Worldings, she writes, "are incipient trajectories [that can] become recognizable as worlds, often with surprise, to those who come into contact with them and who become something in relation to them."[1] I draw upon Stewart's conceptualization of worlding to emphasize conscious desires of making the world differently than it is said to be. These are important aspects of intervening for peace.

Who can do this worlding work of intervening for peace? The answer, I believe, is anyone. We can turn to specific communities for models to build upon. Two key formations of peace activism may help. The first is what we could call the community of expertise activism and the second experiential activism. In the former category we find groups such as the Union of Concerned Scientists, founded by scientists and students at MIT in 1969, the year that the Vietnam War was at its height and the Cuyahoga River in Cleveland was so polluted with oil-soaked debris that it caught on fire when sparks from a passing train hit the water's surface. The organization was concerned with the misuse of scientific and technical knowledge that fed the war machine with weapons development and that contributed to environmental degradation. Its interest was in cultivating a critical examination of governmental policy about science and technology, directing research money away from military technology and nuclear weapons in favor of supporting research that addressed environmental and social problems and encouraging students to pursue research that would be more humane. Another example of expertise activism is that of Physicians for Social Responsibility, which formed in 1961 in opposition to nuclear weapons testing and proliferation. The group initially documented the damages done by Strontium-90, a highly radioactive waste product of atmospheric nuclear testing, and they used their research to argue for the Limited Nuclear Test Ban Treaty that ended atmospheric nuclear testing. It shared the Nobel Peace Prize in 1985 for its campaign to build public awareness and bring an end to the nuclear arms race. In more recent years the group has turned its attention to the health effects of environmental damage caused by climate change and the proliferation of toxic waste and pollution.

Physicians for Human Rights is another expert-driven organization. Founded in 1986, the group is based on the idea that scientists, physicians, and other health professionals have unique skills that lend credibility to the investigation of human rights violations and mass atrocities. With offices in Boston, New York, and Washington, D.C., the organization advocates for persecuted health workers, torture victims, survivors of sexual violence, and sufferers of excessive force during civil unrest.

Humanitarian medical organizations that provide direct care along with policy advocacy bridge the communities of expert and experiential advocacy. Médecins sans Frontières (Doctors without Borders) is perhaps the most prominent example of this. The transnational nongovernmental organization was founded in France in 1971. Reminiscent of the International Red Cross, MSF is committed to remaining politically neutral and impartial in its treatment of patients wounded in wars, tortured by security forces, or sickened by conflict-related disease. With clinics and hospitals all over the world but mainly in the Global South, MSF prioritizes the Hippocratic oath of providing care without causing harm and ensuring patient confidentiality and informed consent. The group's principles of impartiality and neutrality do not preclude it from speaking out publicly against acts of violence against individuals or groups. MSF "stays with the trouble" through internal critique that arises from situations where the safety of its staff is weighed against the dire needs of patients in war zones.[2]

The community of experiential peace activists differs from groups defined by medical and scientific expertise. This community's modes of discourse, sites of intervention, and activist practices derive from experiences of being formally marginalized from decision-making power about war. Many groups make up this community; I want to highlight just a few that are particularly illustrative of world-making by staying with the trouble. The first is the Women's International League for Peace and Freedom (WILPF).[3] It started in 1915 as a group of women working for peace by nonviolent means and promoting political, economic, and social justice. The initial group of over 1,300 women met in The Hague during World War I to protest the war and to "study, make known, and eliminate the causes of war." Jane Addams was WILPF's first international president. Known for her community-based settlement activism at Hull House in Chicago, for advocacy of women's suffrage and peace, and for cofounding the American Civil Liberties Union, Addams delivered a message from WILPF to President Woodrow Wilson in October 1915. He incorporated nine of WILPF's ideas in his Fourteen Points, which became the basis of a peace program that was used in the 1918 armistice establishing peace with Germany and its allies. Throughout the 1920s and 1930s the group was active in chapters throughout Europe and North America, with over fifty thousand members. The group engaged in peace-building throughout World War II, the Korean War in the 1950s, the wars in Southeast Asia during the 1960s and 1970s, and in the Middle East during the 1990s and 2000s. Now based in Geneva, with an office in New York, it uses international laws and conventions and works with the United Nations to make fundamental changes in the way states conceptualize and address gender, militarism, peace, and security.

WILPF was dominated by white women and yet was committed to racial diversity. It had difficulty in its early years attracting African American women to join. The historian Joyce Blackwell recounts how the small number of black women members eventually changed the course of WILPF by calling out the violence of racism in the United States and thereby questioning the organization's definitions of peace and freedom.[4] Officially declared wars, they argued, were only one manifestation of state violence. They raised the crucial point that racialized violence stood in the way of freedom for African Americans in Jim Crow America. A feature of women's organizing for peace has been the movement's internal self-reflexivity and its critical capacity to broaden what counts as peace.

Women Strike for Peace (WSP) started as a direct-action group that evolved out of an international protest against atmospheric nuclear testing on November 1, 1961. As many as fifty thousand women protested in various nations on that day. The group agitated for the Nuclear Test Ban Treaty signed by the United States and the Soviet Union in 1963. Members frequently picketed the White House and Pentagon in the 1960s, protesting nuclear weapons and the Vietnam War. They remained active throughout the 1980s and 1990s, protesting the U.S. interventions in Latin America and the Persian Gulf states, working in coalition with WILPF and other war resister groups. WSP intentionally refused to establish an official hierarchy and depended exclusively on volunteerism. Members convened with women from North and South Vietnam during the war, organized boycotts, and counseled draft resisters. The group did not identify as a feminist organization, though in the early 1970s some of its members did, as the feminist movement grew. In January 1969 they joined other parts of the antiwar and women's liberation movements to form the Jeannette Rankin Brigade, named after the first woman elected to Congress, in 1917, in the first all-women's march in Washington, D.C., to protest war. Following the Vietnam War they returned to an original focus, opposing nuclear proliferation. The New York City chapter gained media attention in staged die-ins and demonstrations against Nixon and Wall Street.[5]

Seneca Women's Encampment for a Future of Peace and Justice (also known as Women's Peace Camp) formed in the summer of 1983.[6] Feminist peace activists in the area had done some guerrilla research to discover that the U.S. Army Seneca Depot was preparing to ship Cruise and Pershing II missiles to Europe in the fall of 1983. The Depot was a weapons storage facility in Romulus, New York, located near Seneca Falls, the site of the first Women's Rights Convention in 1848. The women's original protest against this planned shipment evolved into camp building by women volunteers from among the peace activists. From July 4 through Labor Day women gathered from around the United States to camp on land immediately adjacent to the Depot. The land was purchased with the help of some local radical Catholic nuns. The group emphasized the links between political protest, radically democratic decision-making processes, and peace-building. Like Women Strike for Peace, the Women's Peace Camp was nonhierarchical and had a collective structure. It included members of other peace organizations, such as WILPF, WSP, Catholics against Nuclear Arms, the War Resisters League, Women's Pentagon Action, Rochester Peace and Justice, and the Upstate Feminist Peace Alliance. Men were not allowed to join the encampment or participate in protests. No male over the age of twelve was permitted on the main grounds, but men could stay on the front lawn in a designated spot, a point of controversy in the consensus-driven camp. Some locals derisively called its organizers lesbians and vegetarians. The Peace Camp was an experiment in peace-building through political intervention and performative protest. During some protests the activists wore masks, walked slowly, twisting and turning and pulling each other along, sometimes tying themselves with ribbons and yarn to the fence surrounding the Depot. They performed die-ins. Their embodied protest drew public attention as they acted out the sinister ramifications of nuclear weapons. Peace campers developed a multi-issue agenda that linked activism against militarism with opposition to high rates of inflation, unemployment and poverty, personal violence, addiction, abuse in all its forms, and global environmental destruction. It kept going until 1994. The U.S. Army closed the Depot in 1995 in compliance with the Defense Base Closure and Realignment Act of 1990.

The Women's Peace Camp was part of a larger movement of feminist encampments against nuclear weapons proliferation during the 1980s in North America and Europe. These occupations confronted military secrecy with agitprop tactics, eschewing conventional procedures for registering public complaints and instead going straight to the heart of exposing the relations among war, violence, racism, misogyny, homophobia, and environmental destruction. Several years after the army closed the Seneca Depot it was declared a Superfund site by the Environmental Protection Agency. The radical feminist vision embodied by the Women's Peace Camp had foreseen this and, by occupying the land, critically dramatized how war preparedness actually endangered the lives of citizens the nation claimed to be defending.

The Iraq Veterans against the War (IVAW) is a more recent example of experiential activism that is staying with the trouble in peace-making and worlding. It grew out of a concern raised at the 2004 annual convention of Veterans for Peace that a large number of active-duty service people and veterans who were against the war in Iraq felt various pressures to remain silent. IVAW's agenda was farther reaching than mainstream veterans' advocacy groups that claimed political neutrality and concentrated on raising funds for charitable causes. Instead, from its beginning in 2004, IVAW called for an immediate withdrawal of all occupying forces in Iraq, reparations for the human and structural damages Iraq had suffered, an end to the corporate pillaging of Iraq so that Iraqis could control their own lives and futures, and full benefits and adequate mental and physical health care for returning service men and women. The group expanded in 2009 to include veterans of the war in Afghanistan since their issues were essentially the same. Operating in forty-eight states and on bases overseas, the group sees no battlefield solution to terrorism and calls out military occupation as an aggravating factor in creating resentment among occupied peoples. It calls for the right to self-determination for Afghans and Iraqis against the prolonged occupation of regions over which the United

States, Russia, and China are competing for control of oil and natural gas resources. In 2016 IVAW's board of directors consisted of two women veterans who both enlisted in the military at the age of seventeen and became politicized through their experiences in the military.[7] A majority of the IVAW membership are men, reflecting the demographics of the military, but many women veterans are active in the group. One of its leading campaigns is Operation Recovery, a project aimed at ending the practice of redeploying service members with PTSD, TBI, and military sexual trauma. The campaign addresses the problem of commanding officers overriding the advice of medical professionals and sending traumatized men and women back to active duty. Demanding the right to heal, this campaign links a critique of war-generated suffering with political criticism of imperial wars of occupation and resource stealing.

Tomas Young was a member of the IVAW who in April 2013 announced that he would end his life by refusing his medicine and removing his feeding tube. Young had enlisted in the army immediately after the attacks of September 11, 2001. At twenty-four in 2004 he deployed to Iraq and was severely injured by an IED, resulting in lower-body paralysis and persistent pain. He eventually became a quadriplegic due to medical complications. Before his death Young toured the United States speaking out against the war, disillusioned by the realization that it had been waged on false pretenses. While his story gained some attention in social media and from the circulation of the documentary film *Body of War*, Young's repudiation of the war and of U.S. empire, coupled with the visibility of his anguish and pain, made him a subject unworthy of the biomedical salvation narrative that dominated media coverage about the relationship between war and biomedicine.[8] But for the IVAW and other veterans' peace organizations, Young is remembered as a crucial voice in opposing the seemingly endless wars waged in the name of ridding the world of terrorism that have damaged so many bodies and communities.

The movements, organizations, and activists I have briefly outlined offer perspectives for loosening attachments to war and for living in and with a different ethic of care. By studying these perspectives we may nurture different worlding practices that neither long for a return to some edenic past nor claim that an awful past can be overcome and the future made better by techno-fixes. Dread of an apocalyptic future does not help either; it paralyzes and prevents engagement in world-making practices. Staying with the trouble, as Haraway writes, means being truly present and being responsive and response-able to each other as living beings on a deeply damaged planet. We cannot leave it only to the scientific experts or to the ethical physicians, the peace campers, or activist veterans to make the world we need. Cultivating the ability to respond to one another in troubling times is vital. This means all of us. Our response-ability may loosen ties to war and open up new ways of living and dying together.

I have suggested that one way of undoing the ties between patriotic nationalism and the fetishization of injury and sacrifice is to observe when and where injuries are deemed significant and when and where they are not. A peace-making and worlding practice is paying attention to the instances and contexts when signature wounds appear. On whose bodies are wounds worthy of care? Which bodies bear significant injuries? The response is not to broaden whose injuries get to count as significant but rather to engage in worlding practices in which intentionally inflicted injuries are neither fetishized nor ignored but ended.

I have also questioned the technological salvationism that animates the biomedicine-war nexus. Technical solutions alone are inadequate for contending with problems that need different visions and practices of world-making. Some wounds can be treated by novel biomedical techniques, but what technologies do we have to de-escalate the boiling resentment of occupied people who resort to improvised explosive devices to register their rage against occupiers? What if we imagined replacing the destroy-and-build logic I described with world-making practices oriented toward intervening in institutions and military doctrine that assume salvation must entail the ongoing expendability of life? What if we put the earth's living beings and the environments that sustain them above profits for the few? What if we dethrone the prophets of salvation and doom to cultivate peace in the multidimensional present? Rather than cling to tales of redemption or regenesis that are premised on an original instance of violence in order to generate positive futures, what if we imagined and lived through world-making and peace-making practices that enable the world's many inhabitants to do more than merely survive? What if biomedical researchers and engineers did not have to torque their research interests in order to appeal to military funders? What if they raised their voices against the dogma that war is hell but good for science? What if they said no novel device or therapy should depend for its creation on the steady stream of severely wounded bodies that come home from war? These acts of resistance would be part of the peace-making and worlding I am envisioning.

Attachments are relational. The psychoanalysts who authored attachment theory observed that emotional well-being is an achievement forged in a process of feeling connected and supported by others. When one becomes attached to war, I've argued, the result is a haunting residue of insecurity born of antagonism and an internalized sense of impending threat. These attachments operate within a dualistic arrangement where friend is differentiated from foe and an appropriate response is to be self-protective and suspicious of the other. The Global War on Terror embodies a rhetoric that blends antagonism, suspicion, and fear into a twenty-first-century iteration of nativism, racism, and the exaltation of freedom to dominate other living beings in the name of national defense and imperial benevolence. The blowback from earlier American imperial ventures is ongoing. We need a different world-making ethic of care for what sustains life beyond a vision of free-market-friendly self-improvement and the hope that someday, if we pray long and hard enough, the cycle of violence will magically end. Instead of being attached to war and biomedical salvation, what about caring for peace? I envision peace neither as quietude, banal consensus, nor merely the absence of killing. It is instead an orientation toward response-ability in everyday actions committed to ending violence.

While researching material that went into writing this book I realized that, in many ways, what I was dealing with was a labyrinth of excuses that have been made to rationalize technologically sophisticated violence and the massive devastation it causes. What I discovered is that biomedicine, as both an epistemological formation and an industry, performs an ideological function of bringing war into the realm of the humane through its promises of care and benevolence. In this respect it forges and mobilizes an array of attachments of cruel optimism. It is enlisted to display what can be salvaged from profound destruction, what can be transformed into value from the ruins, and what can be gained in terms of money and knowledge. My intervention has been aimed at exposing the biomedical logics through which we are attached to war, often in ways that are hiding in plain sight, so that we will quit accepting excuses for catastrophic destruction and, as the lyric goes, "lay down the sword and shield . . . and study war no more."[9] It is something I believe we cannot afford not to do.

NOTES

INTRODUCTION

1   Richard Cheney, interviewed by Tim Russert on *Meet the Press*, March 27, 2003.

2   Foucault, *Lectures at the Collège de France*, vol. 3; Mbembe, "Necropolitics."

3   Following Rebecca Solnit, I use the term *citizen* here to mean members of a community, not necessarily limited to those holding legal citizenship (*A Paradise Built in Hell*, 2).

4   Grewal, *Transnational America*; Kaplan and Grewal, "Transnational Practices and Interdisciplinary Feminist Scholarship"; Nordstrom, *Shadows of War*.

5   The gap between U.S. defense spending and that of other nations with large militaries widened with the collapse of the Soviet Union in 1991. In 2011 the U.S. budget reached its peak of $720 billion, edging ahead of the combined amount of comparable defense budgets for the next nineteen highest-spending nations, at $718 billion. While by 2014 the United States had decreased its defense budget to $581 billion and the next highest spenders combined rose to $588 billion, financial analysts noted that the United States would remain the leading spender on defense in the world for the "foreseeable future." See Eastman and McGerty, "Analysis."

According to a 2007 Henry J. Kaiser Foundation report, "Snapshots: Health Care Spending in the United States and Selected OECD Countries," per capita health care spending in the United States increased from $356 in 1970 to $6,697 in 2005 to around $7,500 in 2008. In 2008, 16 percent of the gross domestic product of the United States was devoted to health care spending, compared to 11.2 percent in France, the country with the next greatest share of GDP spending on health. The report compared health care spending in the United States to that of fifteen other countries that ranked in the top three-fifths of per capita national income and aggregate national income. In order of the greatest rate of annual per capita spending to the lowest among these countries in 2008: United States ($7,538), Norway ($5,003), Switzerland ($4,627), Canada ($4,079), Netherlands ($4,063), Austria ($3,970), Germany ($3,737), France ($3,696), Belgium ($3,677), Sweden ($3,470), Australia ($3,353), United Kingdom ($3,129), Spain ($2,902), Italy ($2,870), and Japan ($2,729). Reasons for rising costs in the United States included the expense of new imaging technology; new surgical procedures for replacing faulty organs and joints; new electronic medical records systems and the rise of costly drugs for treating heart disease (the leading cause of death in the United States); the high cost of caring for babies born preterm; the expense of treating long-term chronic illnesses such as HIV/AIDS, diabetes, and renal disease; the rising prices of proprietary pharmaceutical products; and the cost of treatment for an increasing population of substance addicts.

A 2013 report by the Commonwealth Fund (Lorber, "Better Care at Lower Cost") found that the cost of health care per person in the United States annually was $9,200, with an annual total of $2.9 trillion. The average cost for a day in a hospital in the United States was $4,287, while in France it was $853. The price for a normal birth in the United States was $10,000, while in the United Kingdom it was $2,651. A knee replacement in the United States was $25,000, double that of Switzerland. Doctors' visits, drugs, and lab tests were more expensive in the United States than in other developed nations. Despite this, compared to many other developed nations the United States had a higher infant mortality rate, a lower life expectancy, and a greater number of preventable deaths if timely and appropriate treatments were available. The author laid some of the blame for high costs on the fee-for-service arrangement that allows physicians and health management organizations to be paid even if the service (an office visit, test, or treatment) is not effective. Physicians' fear of malpractice may make them inclined to do more tests and procedures. In addition, medical care in the United States is very poorly coordinated between primary physicians and specialists and when moving in and out of hospitals. Sometimes patients with chronic conditions get multiple lab tests that are not needed, or their medications are not adequately coordinated, leading to further problems.

6   Wound ballistics, a field of study that emerged during World War II, is an earlier example of this mutual provocation between war and medicine. According to several of the field's founders, wound ballistics is a study of the mechanics of wounding. It had two main concentrations. First, it studied the factors involved in an injury and the relation between the severity of the wound and the characteristics of the missile or bullet or bomb that caused it (such as its mass, velocity, shape, momentum, and power). The effort was to determine what property of the weapon was most effective in either killing or wounding. Would its fragmentation be most effective? Or its speed? The focus was on the attack. A second aspect of wound ballistics involved the study of the nature of the damage to tissues caused by various aspects of ballistics, including the distance of bullet path, pressure effects of bombs, and tissue stretching caused by a projectile. The close study of a wound and the conditions under which it was sustained would be useful for surgeons in removing dead tissue and debridement necessary for proper recovery. The focus was on healing. "The knowledge of wound ballistics is, therefore, important not only in offense but also in defense," wrote Harvey et al. in "Mechanism of Wounding" (144), based on research they conducted with funding from the Committee on Medical Research, the Office of Scientific Research and Development, and Princeton University between 1943 and 1945.

7   Foucault, *The Birth of the Clinic.*

8   Hall, "Cultural Studies and Its Theoretical Legacies."

9   Hubbard, "Science, Facts, and Feminism," 125.

10 Haraway, "The Promises of Monsters," 295; Haraway, "A Cyborg Manifesto."

11 Masco, *The Theater of Operations*, 37.

12 Masco, *The Theater of Operations*, 73.

13 Both Bowlby and his student and colleague Mary Ainsworth were influenced by Anna Freud and Dorothy Burlingham's wartime research on British children separated from their parents during the Nazi Blitz. Freud and Burlingham noticed that children in residential nurseries exhibited bizarre behavior (sucking their thumbs obsessively, rocking constantly, banging their heads against floors and walls) in order to draw attention to themselves. See Bowlby, "The Nature of the Child's Tie to His Mother"; *Separation Anxiety and Anger*; "Grief and Mourning in Infancy and Early Childhood"; *Attachment and Loss*, vol. 1; and his report to the World Health Organization, *Maternal Care and Mental Health*; Freud and Burlingham, *Infants without Families.*

14 Kaplan, "Precision Targets"; Kaplan et al., "Precision Targets"; Enloe, "How Do They Militarize a Can of Soup?"

15 I am guided in this line of thinking by the work of critical theorists who probe the kinds of affective attachments that tie the personal to the political, taking into consideration especially how the experience of loss generates these ties. The most influential of these for me are Berlant, *Cruel Optimism*; Hartman, *Lose Your Mother*; Love, *Feeling Backward*; Muñoz, *Cruising Utopia*; Sedgwick, *Touching Feeling*; Stewart, *Ordinary Affects.*

16 Berlant, "On Citizenship and Optimism."

17 U.S. Department of Veterans Affairs, Office of Public and Intergovernmental Affairs, "VA Conducts Nation's Largest Analysis of Veteran Suicide."

18 "For Suicidal Veterans, a Frayed Lifeline," *New York Times*, July 16, 2016, accessed July 17, 2016, http://www.nytimes.com/2016/07/17/opinion/sunday/for-suicidal-veterans-a-frayed-lifeline.html?ref=opinion; Leo Shane III and Patricia Klime, "New VA Study Finds 20 Veterans Commit Suicide Each Day," *Military Times*, July 7, 2016, accessed July 17, 2016, http://www.militarytimes.com/story/veterans/2016/07/07/va-suicide-20-daily-research/86788332/.

19 E.H. in comment thread following Lawrence, "At Bagram, War's Tragedy Yields Medical Advances."

20 Conover, "Bullets vs. Band-Aids."

21 On creative destruction, see Schumpeter, *Capitalism, Socialism, and Democracy*, 83. On disaster capitalism, see Klein, *The Shock Doctrine*; Adams, *Markets of Sorrow, Labors of Faith*; Gunewardena and Schuller, *Capitalizing on Catastrophe.*

22 Bush paraphrased these statements on many occasions, but for the first portion of the quote, see Bush, "State of the Union Address"; for the second portion ("I believe there is an Almighty" etc.), see Bush, "Landon Lecture."

23 Bruce Lincoln analyzes Bush's speeches and identifies Christian right-wing phrases and syntax in his discussions of foreign policy in *Holy Terrors.*

24 Nguyen, *The Gift of Freedom*.

25 Disability pay for veterans is an entitlement program, like Medicare and Social Security. A 2007 report issued by the Harvard Kennedy School warned that the budgetary costs of providing compensation benefits and medical care to veterans returning from Iraq and Afghanistan over the course of their lives was estimated to be from $350 billion to $700 billion, depending on the length of deployment, the rate at which they claim disability benefits, and the growth rate of benefits and health care inflation. The figure was based on the 1.4 million U.S. service members who had been deployed to the Global War on Terror between November 2001 and November 2006, of which an estimated 700,000 new patients would enter the VA system. By January 2007, 11 percent of the 24 million living veterans from all wars dating back to World War I were receiving disability benefits. In 2005 the United States paid $23.4 billion in annual disability entitlement pay to veterans from wars preceding the wars in Afghanistan and Iraq. Disability compensation is based on the degree of a veteran's disability on a scale of 0 to 100 percent, with annual benefits ranging from a low of $1,304 per year for a veteran with a 10 percent rating to about $44,000 in annual benefits for those who are completely disabled, though they are also eligible for additional benefits and pensions if severely disabled. An average benefit is $8,890. Veterans receive the compensation benefit for the remainder of their lives once they have been deemed eligible. The average age of service members is twenty-five, so, given a conservatively estimated life expectancy of sixty-five years, the period of compensation could be up to forty years. As of January 2007 the Veterans Benefits Administration had a backlog of 400,000 claims, with an average waiting time of six months to process an original claim and almost two years to process an appeal. See Bilmes, "Soldiers Returning from Iraq and Afghanistan."

26 For an account of the failure of the Department of Veterans Affairs to adequately address U.S. veterans' health care needs following a $15 billion congressional bill, passed in 2014, see David Philipps, "Did Obama's Bill Fix Veterans' Health Care? Still Waiting," *New York Times*, August 5, 2016, accessed August 8, 2016, http://www.nytimes.com/2016/08/06/us/veterans-health-care.html.

27 High rates of unemployment and homelessness among veterans are telling indicators of the disparity between the benefits promised to servicemen and -women and the realities many of them face after leaving the military. Homelessness is particularly acute among African American veterans, who made up only 11 percent of all veterans but accounted for nearly 50 percent of homeless veterans in 2008 (National Alliance to End Homelessness, "Vital Mission," 4). According to the Department of Housing and Urban Development, as of December 2011 approximately 14 percent of all homeless adults were veterans. During a single-night survey in January 2011, more than 67,000 homeless veterans were counted (U.S. Department of Housing and Urban Development, Office of Community Planning and Development, "The 2011 Point-in-Time Estimates of Homelessness"). In 2011 the U.S. Bureau of Labor Statistics reported

that 30.2 percent of veterans between the ages of eighteen and twenty-four were unemployed. The Vocational Rehabilitation and Employment Program of the Veterans Administration provided career counseling and training to over 107,000 veterans with service-related disabilities during 2011 (U.S. Department of Veterans Affairs, "Annual Benefits Report Fiscal Year 2012"). During the twelve months of 2010, over 968,000 veterans between the ages of eighteen and sixty-four were living in poverty (U.S. Department of Commerce, Census Bureau, "Age by Veteran Status by Poverty Status in the Past 12 Months by Disability Status for the Civilian Population 18 Years and Over"). In 2012, 1,000 military families were receiving food stamps. By 2013 the number had grown to 5,000, when the Department of Defense announced that it would no longer award food stamps (Sisk, "DoD: 5,000 Military Families Losing Food Stamps").

28 Farmer, *Infections and Inequalities*; Farmer, *Pathologies of Power*; Abraham, *Mama Might Be Better Off Dead*; Marmot and Wilkinson, *Social Determinants of Health*.

29 Perez-Rivas, "Bush Vows to Rid the World of 'Evil-Doers.'"

30 Hagopian et al., "Mortality in Iraq Associated with the 2003–2011 War and Occupation."

31 Crawford, "Civilian Death and Injury in Afghanistan."

32 Order 81, paragraph 66 (B and C), issued 2002, analyzed in Lea, *Property Rights, Indigenous People and the Developing World*, 268–69.

33 The U.S. military offered discretionary "condolence payments" capped at $2,500 as "expressions of sympathy" but "without reference to fault," as well as "compensation payments" that varied depending on an assessment of claims reviewed by the Department of Defense. A 2007 ACLU study of files acquired through a Freedom of Information Request Act request revealed that, of the 496 files it received, 479 came from Iraq and 17 from Afghanistan. The cases from Iraq ranged from early 2003 to late 2006, with the majority from 2005. The claims from Afghanistan dated mostly from 2006, with one dating back to 2001. Of the 496 files acquired, 198 were denied because the reviewer determined that the incidents arose "from action by an enemy or resulted directly or indirectly from an act of the armed forces of United States in combat" (referred to as "combat exclusion"). About half of the 164 incidents where the United States provided cash "compensation payments" to family members were accompanied by the United States accepting responsibility for the civilian death. The other half received the $2,500 discretionary condolence payment. One case involved an attack with more than a hundred rounds fired on a sleeping family in Iraq that killed the claimant's mother, father, and brother and thirty-two of the family's sheep. The survivor was paid $11,200 and a $2,500 condolence payment. A nine-year-old Iraqi boy was playing outside when a stray bullet killed him; his family was paid $4,000. Source: ACLU, "ACLU Releases Files on Civilian Casualties in Afghanistan and Iraq."

34 See Becker, "Health as Human Capital." Making an argument for investments in education, as these produce more productive people who, he says, are more

likely to be healthy and live longer, Becker calculates that the estimated statistical value of life ranges from $2 million to $9 million for a young person in the United States, with most being between $3 million and $5 million. This is based on an average income of $40,000 a year from 1,900 annual working hours. Adjusting for the other hours during which the individual spends time sleeping or engaging in leisure activities that enhance life and increase the duration of productive life, the adjusted full income is about $220,000 per year. At an annual discount of 5 percent (for the gradual decrease in productive years), the statistical value of a life is about $4.4 million. "This figure," Becker writes, "is not earnings alone but also includes the amount a person is willing to pay to reduce the chances of dying (thus not just lost earning but lost utility that also includes the value of leisure time, and the differences between average and marginal utilities" (385). At $40,000 earnings per year discounted at 5 percent annually, "the present value of the lost earnings from early death is about $1 million, less than a fourth of my back of the envelope estimate of $4.4 million. Therefore, the vast majority of statistical value of life comes not from foregone earnings, but from the loss of leisure time, and differences between average and marginal utilities" (385). Becker is dealing with statistical aggregates, not individual people, but the implications of his calculations are significant: for societies and communities whose educational systems are faltering or destroyed and who have few employment opportunities and even less stress-free time due to massive violent destabilization, the value of a life is calculated at much less than the average for educated members of a stable society with employment opportunities. By these calculations, internally displaced people such as the many Iraqi physicians, despite being educated and employed prior to the U.S. invasion of Iraq, suddenly were worth less with the onset of war.

35 Murphy, "Economization of Life: Calculative Infrastructures of Population and Economy." See also Murphy, "Economization of Life: A Conversation with Leopold Lambert and Michelle Murphy."

36 Murphy, "Economization of Life: A Conversation with Leopold Lambert and Michelle Murphy."

37 Benanav and Clegg, "Misery and Debt."

38 I borrow the trope of scapes from Appadurai, "Disjuncture and Difference in the Global Cultural Economy."

39 Clarke et al., "Biomedicalization."

1 / THE BIOMEDICINE-WAR NEXUS

1 Park, "Morale and the News," 360–61.

2 Bush, *Science, the Endless Frontier*, 17, emphasis added.

3 Eisenhower, "Farewell Address to the Nation," emphasis added.

4 Orr, "The Militarization of Inner Space."

5 Masco, *The Theater of Operations*.

6   Masco, *The Theater of Operations*, 37.

7   Foucault, *Lectures at the Collège de France*, 4:7.

8   Jayadev, "Estimating Guard Labor," 2.

9   Kaplan, "Precision Targets"; Magnet, *When Biometrics Fail*.

10 Bush, "State of the Union Address," 2002.

11 Priest and Arkin, *Top Secret America*.

12 Grewal, "Racial Sovereignty and 'Shooter' Violence."

13 U.S. Department of Homeland Security, "If You See Something, Say Something™."

14 Elbe, "Bodies as Battlefields."

15 For short ethical commentaries on physicians' involvement in force-feeding, see Annas, "Hunger Strikes at Guantanamo"; Crosby et al. "Hunger Strikes, Force-Feeding and Physicians' Responsibilities." On using medicine to inflict torture, see, for example, U.S. Army, Center for Army Lessons Learned, "Commander's Guide to Biometrics in Afghanistan." See also Public Intelligence, "Identity Dominance."

16 See, especially, historical scholarship on disease control, military defense planning, and imperialism in Bashford, *Medicine at the Borders*; Bashford, *Imperial Hygiene*; Bashford and Hooker, *Contagion*; Anderson, *Colonial Pathologies*; McNeill, *Mosquito Empires*; Levien, *Prostitution, Race, and Politics*.

17 Compare, for example, Kristol and Kagan, "Toward a Neo-Reaganite Foreign Policy," explaining the Bush administration's strategy for Afghanistan and Iraq, with Nye, "Get Smart," which defines smart power, a central principle in Obama's foreign policy strategy.

18 Bell, "War and the Allegory of Medical Intervention."

19 Forte, "The Human Terrain System and Anthropology."

20 Bell, "Hybrid Warfare and Its Metaphors," 226.

21 Bell, "War and the Allegory of Medical Intervention," 326.

22 U.S. Army and Marine Corps, *Counterinsurgency: Field Manual 3-24*.

23 All quoted material in this paragraph is from U.S. Army and Marine Corps, *Counterinsurgency: Field Manual 3-24*, chapter 5.2, p. 104.

24 Kilcullen, *The Accidental Guerrilla*, 35–38, 112.

25 Bell, "War and the Allegory of Medical Intervention," 327.

26 McBride and Wibben, "The Gendering of Counterinsurgency in Afghanistan."

27 Fanon, *A Dying Colonialism*, 37–38.

28 Khalili, "The New (and Old) Classics of Counterinsurgency."

29 Khalili, "Gendered Practices of Counterinsurgency," 1474.

30 Kilcullen, "Twenty-Eight Articles," emphasis added.

31 Jones, "Woman to Woman in Afghanistan."

32 See Pottinger et al., "Half-Hearted."

33 USMC Major Nina D'Amato interview is quoted in McBride and Wibben, "The Gendering of Counterinsurgency in Afghanistan," 206, 214n47. For an outstanding analysis of security narratives, see Wibben, *Feminist Security Studies*.

34 Benard et al., *Women and Nation-Building*, 13.

35 A succinct discussion of the militarization of clinics in Iraq and Syria is pre-

sented in Dewachi et al., "Changing Therapeutic Geographies of the Iraq and Syrian Wars."

36 Ali et al., "Annual Mortality Rates and Excess Deaths of Children under Five in Iraq."

37 Garfield, "Civilian Mortality after the 2003 Invasion," 877–79.

38 Levy and Sidel, "Adverse Health Consequences of the Iraq War."

39 Amit R. Paley, "Iraqi Hospitals Are War's New 'Killing Fields,'" *Washington Post*, August 30, 2006, accessed March 18, 2014, http://www.washingtonpost.com /wp-dyn/content/article/2006/08/29/AR2006082901680.html.

40 Donaldson et al., "A Survey of National Physicians Working in an Active Conflict Zone." The researchers surveyed Iraqi physicians working in hospital emergency departments across Iraq from December 2008 through August 2009. The 148 physicians who responded came from over fifty hospitals in eleven provinces. In addition to the large percentage that reported being assaulted by patients or their families (80 percent), they reported working under other very stressful conditions. They saw a median of 7.5 patients an hour, with only 19 percent reporting that their emergency departments had adequate physician staffing. Only 3 percent of the respondents had some type of specialized emergency medicine degree, and only 19 percent were aware of an established triage system in their departments.

41 According to an *Iraq Health Update* report, by 2006 an estimated 18,000 of the 34,000 pre-invasion doctors had fled the country; 250 were kidnapped; and 2,000 had been killed. See Reif, "Conflict Fuels Iraqi Health Crisis."

42 "Morbidity and Mortality among Families in Iraq."

43 SIGIR, "January 2006: Quarterly Report to Congress," 4.

44 T. Christian Miller, "U.S. Priorities Set Back Its Healthcare Goals in Iraq," *Los Angeles Times*, October 30, 2005, accessed March 20, 2014, http://articles.latimes .com/2005/oct/30/world/fg-iraqhealth30.

45 World Health Organization and UN Children's Fund, Countdown to 2015.

46 World Health Organization, "Republic of Iraq," 30.

47 "Morbidity and Mortality among Families in Iraq."

48 Médecins sans Frontières / Doctors without Borders, "Special Report." See also Michael, "Too Good to Be True?"

49 Médecins sans Frontières / Doctors without Borders, "Special Report," 9.

50 This estimate is reported in the International Committee of the Red Cross, "ICRC Survey."

51 Kenny, "The Biopolitics of Global Health."

52 Andrew Marszal, "Doctor Who Helped CIA Track bin Laden Still Languishes in Pakistan Jail," *Telegraph* (U.K.), May 2, 2016, accessed August 11, 2016, http:// www.telegraph.co.uk/news/2016/05/02/doctor-who-helped-cia-track-bin-laden -still-languishes-in-pakist/.

53 Smith, "Polio-Related Murders Kill More than Disease Itself."

54 Donald G. McNeil Jr., "CIA Vaccine Ruse May Have Harmed the War on Polio," *New York Times*, July 9, 2012, accessed June 15, 2015, http://www.nytimes

.com/2012/07/10/health/cia-vaccine-ruse-in-pakistan-may-have-harmed-polio
-fight.html?pagewanted=1&ref=donaldgjrmcneil; Donald G. McNeil Jr., "Getting Polio Campaigns Back on Track," *New York Times*, December 24, 2014,
accessed June 15, 2015, http://www.nytimes.com/2012/12/25/health/getting
-polio-campaigns-back-on-track.html?_r=0.

55 "Deans Protest Sham Vaccination Program in Pakistan."

56 Boyd's remarks are quoted in Moisse, "The Lasting Fallout of Fake Vaccination
Programs."

57 Moturi et al., "Progress toward Polio Eradication." See also U.S. Centers for Disease Control and Prevention, "Progress toward Poliomyelitis Eradication."

58 Dewachi et al., "Changing Therapeutic Geographies of the Iraqi and Syrian Wars."

59 Weizman, *The Least of All Possible Evils*, 11–12.

60 Roberts et al., "Mortality before and after the 2003 Invasion of Iraq."

61 Putting a price on grief and life, the U.S. government paid some of the surviving
spouses of Afghan civilians shot by U.S. troops an average of $2,500. Leaked
documents from 2008 and 2010 show that, in some cases, a surviving child
would receive a "condolence gift" of $1,000. By contrast, the government paid a
death gratuity of $100,000 to families of U.S. soldiers killed in Iraq and Afghan-
istan. Though $2,500 is over twice the average annual income in Afghanistan,
$100,000 is under twice the average annual income in the United States, accord-
ing to the International Monetary Fund estimates of gross domestic product
per capita in 2014. However, U.S. military personnel are covered by low-cost
life insurance for up to $400,000 over the death gratuity, an arrangement that
is based on compensating families for lost income of their member. According
to Pentagon officials, the amount paid to Iraqis and Afghans was not meant to
be compensation for lost wages but was a discretionary sum based on "local
customs" concerning distress and loss. A spreadsheet leaked to investigative
journalists with the Thomson Reuters Foundation showed that one Afghan
family was paid as much for the loss of a cow as for the loss of a family member.
Families were required to file claims with the U.S., British, or German authorities, not with an independent court, in part because the payments were seen
as discretionary, not mandated by law. See Kehoe and Shaw, "Spreadsheets List
Prices Paid for an Afghan Life, a Cow, and a Car."

62 Gilbert and Ponder, "Between Tragedy and Farce," 405.

63 Foucault, *The History of Sexuality*, 138.

64 Li, "To Make Live or Let Die?," 67.

2 / PROMISES OF POLYTRAUMA

1 Government sponsors of AFIRM were the U.S. Army Medical Research and Materiel Command, the Office of Naval Research, the Air Force Medical Service,
the Office of Research and Development of the Department of Veterans Affairs,
the NIH, and the Office of the Assistant Secretary of Defense for Health Affairs.

Baptist Medical Center, Wake Forest, "Institute for Regenerative Medicine to Lead National Effort to Aid Wounded Warriors."

2   Adams et al., "Anticipation."

3   See Whitehead, "Display Wounds." A full transcript can be found in "Display Wounds: Rumination of a Vulnerologist." See also Thyrza Goodeve, "No Wound Ever Speaks for Itself," exploring the idea of an articulate wound.

4   For a discussion of this history, see Terry, "Significant Injury."

5   See Gawande, "Casualties of War." See also Ivey, "Improved Battlefield Triage and Transport May Raise Survival Rates for Severely Wounded Soldiers."

6   U.S. Congressional Budget Office, "The Veterans Health Administration's Treatment of PTSD and Traumatic Brain Injury among Recent Combat Veterans," vii.

7   U.S. Centers for Disease Control and Prevention, "What Are the Signs and Symptoms of Concussion?"

8   "Mild Traumatic Brain Injury: Concussion."

9   See Warden, "Military TBI during the Iraq and Afghanistan Wars." See also DePalma et al., "Blast Injuries," 1341.

10 DePalma et al., "Blast Injuries," 1338. See also Lehman, "Mechanisms of Injury in Wartime."

11 The patent (US 7998290 B2) is held by inventors with Lockheed Martin, acquired through a government contract and published on August 16, 2011. For an explanation of the patent and enhanced blast explosives, see "Enhanced Blast Explosive," *Patents*, accessed August 16, 2016, https://www.google.com/patents /US7998290.

12 According to Colonel Steve Waxman, a U.S. Army physician at the Brooke Army Medical Center in San Antonio, genitourinary trauma accounted for 1 in 20 of the 50,000 combat-related injuries from the beginning of the war in Afghanistan through 2012. Most were penetrating injuries caused by IEDs (29 percent scrotal injury; 9 percent testis; 14 percent penis). Waxman analyzed the files of patients requiring surgery for injuries to their external genitalia at a Combat Support Hospital in Iraq during the troop surge of 2007. Of the 3,595 patients with trauma injuries during those seven months, 1,680 were admitted to the CSH. Ten percent of these (168 patients) had one or more urological injuries, and 115 had one or more injuries to their external genitalia, all caused by fragments from explosions or bullets. See Waxman, "War and Male Genital Trauma"; Waxman et al., "Penetrating Trauma to the External Genitalia in Operation Iraqi Freedom." See also Serkin et al., "Combat Urologic Trauma in U.S. Military Overseas Contingency Operations."

13 Drury, *Signature Wound*.

14 A DCBI Task Force reported that the most dramatic changes that occurred in 2010 in Afghanistan were increased cases of bilateral thigh amputations, triple and quadruple amputations, and associated genital injuries. To put these surge-related injuries in perspective, in 2009, prior to the surge, 274 U.S. service members were killed in Afghanistan and 2,108 were wounded. The numbers for

2010, following the troop surge, were 332 killed in action and 5,095 wounded. According to a lengthy report issued in 2011 by the DCBI Task Force and presented to the U.S. Army Surgeon General, multiple amputations of U.S. service members rose dramatically in Afghanistan in late 2010. The rate of double amputations (both legs amputated) for soldiers and marines evacuated from Afghanistan to Landstuhl Regional Medical Center in Germany increased from 19 percent to 75 percent over the last four months of 2010. Genital injury rates among evacuated soldiers and marines soared from 4 to 11 percent in the last seven months of 2010. U.S. Army, Dismounted Complex Blast Injury Task Force, Report, 5–6.

15 Edwards et al., "Blast Injury in Children." The Injury Severity Score is a method developed in the 1970s for characterizing patients with multiple injuries and designed to assist clinicians in evaluating emergency care. It divides the body into six regions or systems (head and neck, face, chest, abdomen, extremity, external) and uses a scoring system to calculate the overall score for a patient with multiple injuries. See Baker et al., "The Injury Severity Score."

16 Haskell, "Post-deployment Health of OEF/OIF Women Veterans Who Use VA." Between 2003 and 2010 twenty-six servicewomen were admitted to the four leading polytrauma VA hospitals in the United States, compared with over 350 servicemen admitted between 2001 and 2007. U.S. Department of Veterans Affairs, "Frequently Asked Questions." Of the 327,633 veterans of Operation Enduring Freedom in Afghanistan and Operation Iraqi Freedom who were screened for traumatic brain injury, 287,185 were men and 40,448 were women (women composed around 15 percent of service members in all branches combined). Of these, mild TBI was confirmed in 11,951 of the men and 654 of the women. Iverson, "Clinical and Methodological Challenges with Assessing Mild Traumatic Brain Injury in the Military."

17 To underscore the amount of care that is needed, the VA caregiver stipend was established for those assisting veterans with activities of daily living. Authorized by the FY 2010 National Defense Authorization Act, the Special Compensation for Assistance with Activities of Daily Living "provides monthly compensation for Service members who incur permanent, catastrophic illnesses or injuries in the line of duty that require the services of a home health aide to provide non-medical care, support, and assistance." The program provided up to ninety days of payments after separation from active duty based on the level of care needed and the prevailing rates for home health aides in the geographic area of the service member's residence. The program delineated three tiers of care: high = need for a full-time caregiver who provides forty hours of personal care per week; medium = twenty-five hours a week needed; low = ten hours a week needed. U.S. Army, "Special Compensation for Assistance with Activities of Daily Living (SCAADL)."

18 See U.S. Department of Veterans Affairs, "Polytrauma/TBI System of Care."

19 U.S. Army, Dismounted Complex Blast Injury Task Force, Report, 30.

20 See McCall, "Top 5 Army Medical Innovations."

21 For similar accounts that link regenerative medicine with a promising future for wounded veterans, see Hipp, "How Military Medicine Is Leading the Way"; Klime, "Surgery, Treatments Can Restore Injured Troops' Sexual Function"; Miles, "Regenerative Medicine Shows Promise for Wounded Warriors"; Underwood, "Military Medicine"; Drummond, "World's Most Wired War Healer"; Peet, "Rutgers University Anchors U.S. Military Project in Regenerative Medicine"; Leick, "Stem Cells and Regenerative Medicine Help Kansans."

22 "Growing Body Parts."

23 Cooper, *Life as Surplus*, 142, 144.

24 See Williams, "Five Unlikely Companies Bucking the Biotech Sell-Off."

25 For a colorful account of Atala's involvement in the debate over the use of human embryonic stem cells, see Cabot, "Whatever Happened to Stem Cells?"

26 Piore and Lewis, "How Pig Guts Became the Next Bright Hope for Regenerating Human Limbs."

27 Between September 18 and October 9, 2001, four envelopes containing anthrax spores were sent anonymously to the *New York Post*, NBC anchorman Tom Brokaw, Senator Tom Daschle, and Senator Patrick Leahy. The Centers for Disease Control confirmed that twenty-three people contracted anthrax from contact with these envelopes, seventeen were sickened, and five died. For the FBI's account of the attacks, see FBI, "Amerithrax or Anthrax Investigation."

28 Piore and Lewis, "How Pig Guts Became the Next Bright Hope for Regenerating Human Limbs."

29 Piore and Lewis, "How Pig Guts Became the Next Bright Hope for Regenerating Human Limbs."

30 Anderson, "Marine Wounded Warrior Offered Bittersweet Opportunity."

31 Seth Messinger posits two models of rehabilitation based on his fieldwork as an embedded anthropologist from July 2006 to January 2008 in the U.S. Armed Forces Amputee Patient Care Program at Walter Reed Army Medical Center. The first and dominant one is a sports model that emphasizes physical functioning in which the ideal patient is someone who will listen to the coach. The second model, evident in how patients responded "idiosyncratically" to the sports model, emphasized what Messinger calls a refashioning of identity in relation to the meaning of injury and patients' ideas about the future. He writes, "Patients face several disruptions as a result of their limb-loss and world making is an important aspect of their more personal notions of what constitutes recovery. This, more personal, focus on recovery could fit well with the overall program goals, but often put patients at a remove, or at cross-purposes, with their therapists and physicians and was a tension which could have potentially negative implications in terms of how patients were evaluated." Messinger, "Medical Anthropology in a Military Treatment Facility." See also Messinger, "Getting Past the Accident"; Wool, "On Movement"; Wool, *After War*.

32 Ticktin, *Casualties of Care*, 19, 204, emphasis added. See also Mouffe, *On the Political*; Rancière, *Dissensus*.

33   Bush, "President Discusses Stem Cell Research."

34   See Bush, Executive Order 13435.

35   For an account of the tensions between public funding for social justice in health care and stem cell research in the state of California, see Benjamin, *People's Science*.

36   White House, "Remarks of President Barack Obama as Prepared for Delivery Signing of Stem Cell Executive Order [EO 13505] and Scientific Integrity Memorandum."

37   O'Brien, "The Great Stem Cell Dilemma."

38   The 2011 Annual Report of AFIRM states that between 2008 and 2011 about $100 million of the total $300 million funding came from the U.S. government (army, navy, air force, VA, NIH); $80 million came from matching funds from state governments and participating universities; $109 million came from pre-existing research projects directly related to deliverables of the AFIRM from the NIH, DARPA, congressional special programs, the NSF, and philanthropy; and $25 million from the Defense Health Program.

39   Subordinate commands of the USAMRMC are in Natick, Mass.; Aberdeen, Md.; Fort Rucker (Alabama); Fort Sam Houston (Texas); Walter Reed Army Institute of Research in Silver Spring, Md.; Crystal City, Va.; Kenya (research unit focused on predicting, detecting, and preventing infectious disease threats to military and civilians in East Africa); Heidelberg and Pirmasens (Germany); Camp Carroll (Korea); Bangkok (focus on epidemiology of "military-important diseases endemic to tropical regions"); and at the Dover Air Base in Dover, Del., at the U.S. armed forces morgue facility, which focuses on forensic pathology, forensic toxicology, DNA technology, and identification and mortality surveillance.

40   From the Telemedicine and Advanced Technology Research Center website, accessed April 23, 2014, http://www.tatrc.org.

41   The Rutgers/Cleveland Clinic Consortium included scientists, physicians, and bioengineers from Brigham and Women's Hospital in Boston, Carnegie Mellon University, Case Western Reserve University, Cooper Medical School of Rowan University, Dartmouth Medical School and School of Engineering, Massachusetts General Hospital, Harvard Medical School, Massachusetts Institute of Technology, the Mayo Clinic, Northwestern University, State University of New York at Stony Brook, the University of Cincinnati, the University of Medicine and Dentistry of New Jersey, Vanderbilt University, and the Universities of Michigan, Pennsylvania, and Virginia. The Wake Forest–Pittsburgh Consortium included researchers from the McGowan Institute, the Wake Forest Institute for Regenerative Medicine, Georgia Institute of Technology, Johns Hopkins Medical School, Rice University, Stanford University, Tufts University, the Oregon Medical Laser Center, and the multicampus Institute for Collaborative Biotechnologies (UC Santa Barbara, MIT, California Institute of Technology).

42   Industry partners listed in AFIRM's 2011 Annual Report are Arteriocyte, Avita Medical, Axonia Medical, Biologics Consulting Group, Biosafe-America, BioStat

International, BonWrx, Cynvenio Biosystems, Fidia Advanced Biopolymers (Italy), GID Group, Glycosan BioSystems, Healthpoint Biotherapeutics/DFB Bioscience, ImageIQ, Integra Spine/Integra Life Sciences, Kensey Nash Corporation, KeraNetics, Lexmark, LifeCell Corporation, LifeNet Health, Lonza Walkersville, Maricopa Integrated Health Systems, MedDRA Assistance, Medtronic, Neodyne Biosciences, Nitinol Development Corporation, NOVOTEC, Organogenesis, Osteotech, PeriTec Biosciences, Proxy Biomedical, SimQuest, Stratatech Corporation, Stryker Corporation, Tolera Therapuetics, Trident Biomedical.

43 Adams et al., "Anticipation."

44 Cooper, *Life as Surplus*, 103.

45 Cooper, *Life as Surplus*, 111–13.

46 Andrew Pollack, "Questioning the Allure of Putting Cells in the Bank," *New York Times*, January 29, 2008, accessed May 1, 2014, http://www.nytimes.com /2008/01/29/health/29stem.html?pagewanted=all.

47 Pollack, "Questioning the Allure."

48 Miles, "Regenerative Medicine Shows Promise for Wounded Warriors."

49 AFIRM, "Our Science for Their Healing," in Annual Report, p. 272.

50 Journalist Bob Drury covered the subject in a feature story in *Men's Health* that later was expanded into a Kindle single titled *Signature Wound*. In the short book Drury provides vivid accounts of his conversations with veterans being treated for IED-related genital injuries at VA facilities. His highly sympathetic yet spare prose aims to lift the taboo and shame associated with this particular kind of injury and the toll it takes on the identity and psychological health of its victims. For a similar approach, see David Wood, "Beyond the Battlefield: Afghanistan's Wounded Struggle with Genital Injuries," *Huffington Post*, March 12, 2012, accessed April 30, 2014, http://www.huffingtonpost.com/2012/03/21/beyond-the -battlefield-afghanistan-genital-injuries_n_1335356.html.

51 Chen et al., "Bioengineered Corporal Tissue for Structural and Functional Restoration of the Penis."

52 Baptist Medical Center, Wake Forest, "Scientists Successfully Grow Animal Penile Erectile Tissue in Lab."

53 Quote in Wood, "Beyond the Battlefield."

54 Wood, "Beyond the Battlefield."

55 Wool, *After War*, back cover, 158.

56 Wool, *After War*, 158.

57 Linker, *War's Waste*.

58 Wool, *After War*, 169, 171, emphasis added.

3 / WE CAN ENHANCE YOU

1 Dentzer, "Prosthetic Sculptures Duplicate Faces of Wounded U.S. Soldiers."

2 Herr, "The Double Amputee Who Designs Better Limbs."

3 Quoted in Business Innovation Factory, "Hugh Herr at BIF-2."

4 Tom A. Peter, "Military Inventions Hit the Civilian Market," *Christian Science Monitor*, June 19, 2008, accessed May 29, 2014, http://www.csmonitor.com /Innovation/Tech-Culture/2008/0619/built-for-battle-but-perfect-in-peacetime.

5 Ling is quoted in Miles, "DARPA's Cutting-Edge Programs Revolutionize Prosthetics."

6 Fischer, "A Guide to U.S. Military Casualty Statistics," 2, 7.

7 Berlant, "On Citizenship and Optimism."

8 See, for example, Baudrillard, *The Transparency of Evil*; Hayles, *How We Became Posthuman*; Ronell, *Crack Wars*; Virilio, *The Vision Machine*.

9 Smith and Morra, *The Prosthetic Impulse*, 3.

10 See especially Ott et al., *Artificial Parts, Practical Lives*; Mitchell and Snyderman, *The Body and Physical Differences*; Jain, "The Prosthetic Imagination"; Kurzman, "Performing Able-Bodiedness" and "Presence and Prosthesis."

11 Lukes, "The Sovereignty of Subtraction."

12 Serlin, "Queerness and Disability in U.S. Military Culture." For more on this distinction, see Skocpol, *Protecting Soldiers and Mothers*; Liachowitz, *Disability as a Social Construct*.

13 Garland-Thomson, "Cultural Logic of Euthanasia," 779, 780, 781.

14 Garland-Thomson, "Cultural Logic of Euthanasia," 791.

15 Schweik, *The Ugly Laws*, 150.

16 The Department of Veterans Affairs invested $583 million for medical and prosthetics research in 2013, up from $581 million in 2010, and $580 million each year in 2011 and 2012. Between 2006 and 2014 DARPA spent $144 million on prosthetics research and development. Between 2009 and 2014 DARPA spent $71.2 million of the total $144 million on brain-machine interface neural prosthetic devices. See "The Future of Artificial Limbs."

17 Source for $12.67 billion figure: Markets and Markets, "Medical Bionic Implant / Artificial Organs Market." According to this source, the key players in the business were Biomet, Medtronic, Ekso Bionics, Second Sight Medical Products, and St. Jude Medical, all U.S.-based companies, along with Össur of Iceland; Orthofix International, a Dutch firm; and Cochlear Ltd. of Australia.

18 O'Connor, "'Fractions of Men,'" 767.

19 *Flexibility* is a cherished trope in post-Fordist capitalism. Outsourcing, just-in-time supplying of human and material means of production, horizontal management, and teamwork are its central features. It is often contrasted to unionized labor, in which the worker is protected from mandatory overtime; instead work assignments are contingent. Workers are expected to work on themselves, to improve themselves both on the job and off. Fitness regimes and employee wellness programs emphasize physical and mental fitness in normative terms. *Flexible Bodies*, Emily Martin's important study of the emergence of flexibility in popular discourses about the body's immune system during the rise of the HIV/AIDS epidemic, is relevant here. Martin and her research team discovered

that the immune system was described by scientists, holistic practitioners, and ordinary people as a complex field whose relative flexibility was correlated to health. The growing consensus was that a flexible immune system was better able to handle allergies, heart disease, cancer, and HIV/AIDS than one that could not change swiftly. Martin noticed a corollary in business terminology wherein flexibility and teamwork were valued over the individual. Workers and organizations that could adapt quickly to changing conditions of post-Fordist economies were valued, and those seen as lacking these qualities were less fit for survival. In both immunology and business, flexible bodies were the accomplishments of people who put their minds to being amenable and able to change. The formula worked to the advantage of employers whose workers were required to take on a variety of tasks. It suggested that people with immune disorders could improve their situation by pursuing treatments and techniques to become flexible. Martin referred to the effects of this new elevation of flexible bodies as a form of social Darwinism that was friendly to post-Fordist capitalism. For another valuable source on flexible accumulation, the labor market, and bodies, see Lowe, *The Body in Late-Capitalist USA*.

20 Serlin, *Replaceable You*.

21 Kinsey et al., *Sexual Behavior in the Human Male*.

22 Serlin, *Replaceable You*, 16, 14.

23 Cartwright and Goldfarb, "On the Subject of Neural and Sensory Prostheses."

24 Bennett, *Vibrant Matter*.

25 Crawford, *Phantom Limb*, 3, 4.

26 Alexander, "Rivaling Nature."

27 In May 2009 Siemionow appeared at a press conference with her patient, Connie Culp, several months after the transplant surgery. Culp was forty-six years old at the time. Four years earlier her husband shot her in the face before turning the shotgun on himself. Both of them survived, but his injuries were minor while hers were severe. She lost her nose, one eye, her upper and lower jaw, her palate, and her lower eyelids. Leading up to the transplant surgery, she underwent thirty operations in which doctors removed parts of her ribs to shape cheekbones out of them and used bone from her legs to shape an upper jaw. The transplant surgery took twenty-two hours, part of it to remove the face of the deceased donor who had died of a heart attack and the rest to conduct the microsurgery necessary to connect the nerves and blood vessels of that tissue to the recipient. In just over a month Culp's body began to show signs of rejecting the tissue, so she was treated with steroids. By 2013 she had gained a sense of smell and taste and the nerves in her face had regenerated. Higgs, "Cleveland Clinic Doctors Perform First Almost-Total Face Transplant in the United States." See also Brie Zeltner, "Cleveland Clinic Face Transplant Patient Connie Culp Hopes Her Story Teaches People Not to Judge," *Cleveland Plain Dealer*, May 5, 2009, accessed August 14, 2014, http://www.cleveland.com/medical/index.ssf/2009/05/face_transplant.html.

Surgeons performed a soft tissue transplant on Isabelle Dinoire, a thirty-eight-year-old woman whose dog chewed off the lower part of her face while she was unconscious after taking sleeping pills. The donor was a forty-six-year-old woman who had committed suicide. The surgeons transplanted a mouth, chin, and nose. After months of physical therapy and a continual dosage of antirejection drugs, Dinoire regained some ability to open her mouth to eat, speak, and smile. See Jon Henley and Sarah Boseley, "Dog Attack Victim Gets World's First Face Transplant," *Guardian* (U.K.), November 30, 2005, accessed August 14, 2014, http://www.theguardian.com/science/2005/dec/01/france.medicineandhealth. See also Ariane Bernard and Craig S. Smith, "French Face-Transplant Patient Tells of Her Ordeal," *New York Times*, February 7, 2006, accessed August 14, 2014, http://www.nytimes.com/2006/02/07/international/europe/07face.html?_r=0.

28   On his CV Hanson lists a performance piece from 1994 (accessed August 15, 2014, http://hansonrobotics.files.wordpress.com/2011/11/hansoncv_2011-11 -11.pdf).

29   See David Segal, "This Man Is Not a Cyborg. Yet.," *New York Times*, June 1, 2013, accessed August 15, 2014, http://www.nytimes.com/2013/06/02/business /dmitry-itskov-and-the-avatar-quest.html?pagewanted=all&_r=0.

30   *Mindfiles, Mindware and Mindclones*, accessed March 13, 2017, http://mindclones .blogspot.com/.

31   BINA48 stands for Breakthrough Intelligence via Neural Architecture 48, but also for Bina Aspen Rothblatt, Martine Rothblatt's wife. The humanoid robot was developed based on the compilation of over a hundred hours of Aspen Rothblatt's memories, emotions, and beliefs. The robot is capable of carrying on conversations on the Internet and has sixty-four facial expressions developed by Hanson. BINA48 appeared in a TED Talk in 2012, was interviewed in 2014 by Stephen Colbert on *The Colbert Report*, and appeared in a 2016 episode of the Netflix series *Chelsea Does*, where she had a short conversation with Chelsea Handler.

32   Hanson Robotics, "About Hanson Robotics."

33   Prosthetics research was funded by the Department of Defense's Telemedicine and Advanced Technology Research Center, established in 1998; the Department of Veterans Affairs; DARPA; and the Armed Forces Institute for Regenerative Medicine.

34   The estimate was stated by John R. Fox, the director of the Orthotic and Prosthetic Lab at Hunter Holmes McGuire Veterans Administration Medical Center, and reported in Tammie Smith, "Prosthetic Limbs Get Smarter with Microprocessors," *Richmond (Va.) Times Dispatch*, July 15, 2013, accessed June 24, 2014, http://www.timesdispatch.com/business/health/prosthetic-limbs-get-smarter -with-microprocessors/article_97d5c474-0e9c-5bfa-8ea2-a01dc440590e.html.

35   "The Bionic Man Who Builds Bionic People."

36   For a popular account of Herr's background and accomplishments in prosthetic design, see "The Bionic Man Who Builds Bionic People."

37   Biomechatronics Group, "About."

38   Source: Össur Americas website, accessed June 20, 2014, http://www.ossur.com /americas.

39   The figure of $50,000 was reported in Schwartz, "A Brand-New Kick."

40   See U.S. Army, Medical Department, Brooke Army Medical Center website, accessed June 10, 2014, http://www.bamc.amedd.army.mil/departments /orthopaedic/cfi/; Rawlings, "Where Miracles Are Made."

41   The quote from Herr originally appeared on his website, Personal Bionics, which is no longer functioning. The quote migrated to the BiONX website, accessed February 26, 2017, http://www.bionxmed.com/payer/the-biom-advantage/. Hugh Herr is on the board of directors of the BiONX Company and is listed as the company's founder.

42   Donoghue, "Connecting Cortex to Machines," figure 1.

43   See Cartwright and Goldfarb, "On the Subject of Neural and Sensory Prostheses," 138, emphasis added.

44   Richard Weir worked with Jack Schorsch of the Rehabilitation Institute of Chicago and Philip Troyk, a biomedical engineering professor at the Illinois Institute of Technology, to develop the IMES.

45   Pierce, "Hugh Herr's New Parts"; Venkataramanan, "In Pictures."

46   "The Bionic Man Who Builds Bionic People."

47   For more on the symposium, see MIT Media Lab, "H2.0: New Minds, New Bodies, New Identities."

48   Herr, "The New Bionics That Let Us Run, Climb and Dance."

49   Benjamin Bratton, "We Need to Talk about TED," *Guardian* (U.K.), December 30, 2013, accessed June 27, 2014, http://www.theguardian.com/comment isfree/2013/dec/30/we-need-to-talk-about-ted.

50   Jurgenson, "Against TED."

51   See, for example, Lane, *The Mask of Benevolence*.

52   Much of the scholarly literature that discusses the shortcomings of technological salvationism inherent in the medical model of disability zeroes in on the ethics of prenatal screening. See, for example, Asch, "Appearance-Altering Surgery, Children's Sense of Self, and Parental Love"; Parens and Asch, "Disability Rights Critique of Prenatal Testing"; Rapp, *Testing Women, Testing the Fetus*. See also the critical interventions concerning technological solutions offered in Wolbring, "Disability Rights Approach toward Bioethics"; Shakespeare, *Disability Rights and Wrongs Revisited*. For a compelling critique of how compulsory able-bodiedness and able-mindedness have conceived of time and the future to define disability as a predetermined limit, see Kafer, *Feminist, Queer, Crip*. Kafer draws together ideas from environmental justice, transgender politics, and reproductive justice in arguing for new crip futures and alliances among feminist, queer, and crip movements.

53   According to the *Boston Globe*, the bombs detonated at 2:49 p.m., twelve seconds and 214 yards apart. The bombs, made using pressure cookers, killed three and

wounded 267. Police began a search for two men spotted in surveillance footage in the area, believed to be the ones who planted the bombs in backpacks they dropped off. The suspects were two brothers in their twenties named Dzhokhar and Tamerlan Tsarnaev. Three nights after the bombing a security guard at MIT was killed, a murder that was later tied to the brothers. They then carjacked a hostage at gunpoint who managed to escape and called the police to tell them that the brothers spoke openly about being the bombers. The older brother, Tamerlan, was shot and killed by police in nearby Watertown in the early hours of that third night after the bombing, but Dzhokhar was able to elude the police. The greater Boston area was put on lockdown, and many houses in the Watertown area were searched for all of the fourth day. Once the lockdown was lifted as night fell, a Watertown resident checked his boat and found bloodstains on it. He called the police, who captured Dzhokhar, suffering from gunshot wounds to his head, neck, legs, and hand. He was taken to a local hospital for care and held for indictment. He was sentenced to death by a federal jury on May 15, 2015. Four of the brothers' friends were charged as accomplices for destroying evidence following the bombings. See "Terror at the Marathon," *Boston Globe*, accessed June 27, 2014, http://www.bostonglobe.com/metro/specials/boston-marathon-explosions; Ann O'Neill, Aaron Cooper, and Ray Sanchez, "Boston Marathon Bomber Dzhokhar Tsarnaev Sentenced to Death," *CNN*, May 17, 2015, accessed June 1, 2015, http://www.cnn.com/2015/05/15/us/boston-bombing-tsarnaev-sentence/.

54 Adee, "Winner."
55 DARPA, "DARPA Launches Biological Technologies Office."
56 Beard, "DARPA's Bio-Revolution."
57 Wessberg et al., "Real-Time Prediction of Hand Trajectory by Ensembles in Cortical Neurons in Primates."
58 See Biological Technologies Office, DARPA.
59 "The Pentagon's Bionic Arm."
60 Belfiore, *The Department of Mad Scientists*, 5.
61 Ling quoted in Miles, "Defense Agency Makes Big Advances in Prosthetics Research."
62 Ling quoted in DARPA, "DARPA Launches Biological Technologies Office."
63 DARPA, "From Idea to Market in Eight Years."
64 A study published in 2010 found that among 581 upper-limb amputee veterans and service members surveyed, the 298 who were part of the Vietnam War cohort had a higher rate of prosthetic abandonment (i.e., they quit wearing their devices) compared to the OIF/OEF cohort of 283. Only 70 percent of the Vietnam War cohort used prostheses, and 78 percent of this group used low-tech mechanical devices. The OIF/OEF cohort used prostheses at a rate double that of their Vietnam War counterparts, and of the former cohort, 46 percent used myoelectric devices and 38 percent used low-tech mechanical devices. See Blough et al., "Prosthetic Cost Projections for Servicemembers with Major Limb Loss from Vietnam and OIF/OEF."

65   Robotic upper limbs on the market around 2011 that had these limited capabilities included Dynamic Arm by Otto Bock, Utah Arm by Motion Control, iLimb Hand by Touch Bionics, Boston Arm by LTI, and BeBionic Hand.

66   Kuniholm, "An Open-Source Approach to Better Prosthetics."

67   Kuniholm presented this critique in a 2011 TEDx Talk in Chapel Hill, North Carolina, on the theme "Global Health and Technology." His talk was titled "We Have the Technology, Right?"

68   Kuniholm made these remarks in "An Open-Source Approach to Better Prosthetics" and "We Have the Technology, Right?"

69   See the Open Prosthetics Project website: The Open Prosthetics Project: An Initiative of the Shared Design Alliance, accessed July 1, 2014, http://open prosthetics.org/.

70   See "Marine Captain Jon Kuniholm Speaks @ the 2008 DNC."

4 / PATHOGENIC THREATS

1   U.S. Senate, "Avian Flu Pandemic," S10656. Ultimately the Department of Defense Emergency Supplemental Appropriations to Address Hurricanes in the Gulf of Mexico and Pandemic Influenza Act, 2006, provided $1.17 billion in supplemental funding following Hurricanes Katrina and Rita, of which $94 million was given to the Department of Agriculture for avian influenza activities in preparation for a potential outbreak. For details, see U.S. House of Representatives, "H. Rept. 109-746."

2   U.S. Senate, "Avian Flu Pandemic."

3   For a thorough account and analysis, see Guillemin, *American Anthrax*.

4   Ahuja, *Biosecurities*, 5.

5   On the history of disease control, military defense planning, and imperialism, see Bashford, *Medicine at the Borders*; Bashford, *Imperial Hygiene*; Bashford and Hooker, *Contagion*; Mitropoulos, *Contract and Contagion*, especially her chapter "Unproductive Circulation, Excessive Consumption," 119–34.

6   Masco, *The Theater of Operations*, 150, 146.

7   The full text of Powell's speech to the United Nations on Iraq is "A Policy of Evasion and Deception," *Washington Post*, February 5, 2003, accessed August 1, 2016, http://www.washingtonpost.com/wp-srv/nation/transcripts/powelltext _020503.html. Powell later denounced his testimony in Powell and Koltz, *It Worked for Me*: "A failure will always be attached to me and my U.N. presentation. But I am mad mostly at myself for not having smelled the problem. My instincts failed me." Powell asserted that "there would have been no war" in Iraq had the Bush administration understood that Hussein did not possess any functioning unconventional weapons (223).

8   White House, "The 2003 State of the Union Address."

9   According to the North Carolina Biotechnology Center, by 2015 North Carolina had close to six hundred bioscience companies that directly employed over

sixty thousand people, and another two thousand North Carolina–based companies to support bioscience companies. The Center was established as the first government-sponsored initiative for economic development through biotechnology. The state established it as a nonprofit private corporation in 1984 to provide funding in the form of grants, loans, and other assistance to universities and private companies for research. In 2015 the Center reported nearly $16 million of awards to around ninety companies and helped them raise over $1 billion from other sources. See North Carolina Biotechnology Center, "About Us." As of 2015 several of the world's largest bioscience and pharmaceutical corporations had laboratories in North Carolina, including Archer Daniels Midland, Novartis, Novo Nordisk, Pfizer, Merck, and GlaxoSmithKline, most of them located in Research Triangle Park, which facilitated networking with nearby Duke University, the University of North Carolina at Chapel Hill, and North Carolina State University.

10 Rumsfeld spoke of "known unknowns" and "unknown unknowns" on various occasions: "Reports that say that something hasn't happened are always interesting to me, because as we know, there are known knowns; there are things we know we know. We also know there are known unknowns; that is to say we know there are some things we do not know. But there are also unknown unknowns—the ones we don't know we don't know. And if one looks throughout the history of our country and other free countries, it is the latter category that tend to be the difficult ones." U.S. Department of Defense, News Briefing, Secretary Rumsfeld and General Richard Myers. Several months later, during a press conference at NATO headquarters in Brussels, he stated, "Now what is the message there? The message is that there are known 'knowns.' These are things we know that we know. There are known unknowns. That is to say there are things that we now know we don't know. But there are also unknown unknowns. There are things we do not know we do not know. So when we do the best we can and we pull this information together, and we then say that's basically what we see as the situation, that is really only the known knowns and the known unknowns. And each year, we discover a few more of those unknown unknowns." U.S. Department of Defense, News Transcript, Secretary Rumsfeld Press Conference at NATO Headquarters. Rumsfeld was drawing from a poem by D. H. Lawrence entitled "New Heaven and New Earth," which is itself a spin on Revelation 21:1–6.

11 Adams et al., "Anticipation."

12 Elbe, "Bodies as Battlefields."

13 See, for example, the U.S. Department of Defense's 2010 *Quadrennial Defense Review Report*: "Countries that have the infrastructure and capability to report and track the spread of an outbreak of disease are more able to save more lives. Detecting, diagnosing, and determining the origin of a pathogen will enable U.S. authorities to better respond to future disease outbreaks and identify whether they are natural or man-made. Accordingly, we are expanding the biological

threat reduction program to countries outside the former Soviet Union in order to create a global network for surveillance and response" (36).

14   Lakoff, "Two Regimes of Global Health."

15   Lakoff, "Two Regimes of Global Health," 59.

16   Lakoff, "Two Regimes of Global Health," 60.

17   Lakoff concludes his article by suggesting that, rather than seeing these two regimes as contradictory, they should be seen as complementary: "If so, humanitarian biomedicine could be seen as offering a philanthropic palliative to nation-states lacking public health infrastructure in exchange for the right of international health organizations to monitor their populations for outbreaks that might threaten the wealthy nations" ("Two Regimes of Global Health," 75).

18   Valuable historical accounts of biological warfare are Wheelis et al., *Deadly Cultures*; Geissler and Moon, *Biological and Toxin Weapons*; Guillemin, *Biological Weapons*. See also Rubin, *The Living Weapon*.

19   Mitropoulos, *Contract and Contagion*, 121.

20   Wald, *Contagious*.

21   Fauci and Collins, "Benefits and Risks of Influenza Research."

22   League of Nations, "Protocol for the Prohibition of the Use in War of Asphyxiating, Poisonous or Other Gases."

23   Guillemin, "Scientists and the History of Biological Weapons."

24   For the specific wording of the BTWC, see Arms Control Association, *Biological Weapons Convention*.

25   For more on Ogarkov, see FitzGerald, "Marshal Ogarkov on Modern War." See also Metz and Kievit, "Strategy and the Revolution in Military Affairs."

26   Quoted in Garrett, *Betrayal of Trust*, 541.

27   See White House, "U.S. Policy on Counterterrorism" (PDD/NSC-39), "Protection against Unconventional Threats to the Homeland and Americans Overseas" (PDD/NSC-62), and "Critical Infrastructure Protection" (PDD/NSC-63).

28   Judith Miller, "Company Led by Top Admiral Buys Michigan Lab," *New York Times*, July 8, 1998, accessed June 20, 2015, http://www.nytimes.com/1998/07/08 /us/company-led-by-top-admiral-buys-michigan-vaccine-lab.html.

29   Fuad El-Hibri is quoted in Rozen, "The Anthrax Vaccine Scandal."

30   Keith Bradsher, "A Nation Challenged: The Supplies; The Only U.S. Laboratory for the Anthrax Vaccine Says Production Will Be Delayed," *New York Times Business Day*, November 12, 2001, accessed July 2, 2015, http://www.nytimes .com/2001/11/12/business/nation-challenged-supplies-only-us-laboratory-for -anthrax-vaccine-says.html.

31   The group formed during the Clinton presidency and reported its assessment in Kagan et al., *Rebuilding America's Defenses*. The doctrine of preemption was first explicitly articulated in Bush, "The National Security Strategy of the United States of America."

32   Project for the New American Century, "Letter to Honorable William J. Clinton."

33   U.S. Army, *Field Manual 3-0*, 1–15, 16.

34 Cooper, *Life as Surplus*, 89.

35 Bacher et al., "Anticipatory Evolution and DNA Shuffling."

36 Beginning in 1999 the U.S. Department of Energy sponsored research to build a biodetection system called BASIS (Biological Aerosol Sentry and Information System), developed by scientists at Lawrence Livermore and Los Alamos National Laboratories within the Chemical and Biological Security Program of the Energy Department's Nuclear Security Administration. In early 2003 it was installed in various urban centers. It consists of a portable air collector coupled to a series of filters that capture airborne particles passing through the system. The filter was designed to determine when an attack occurred using sequential filters automatically rotated on an hourly basis. Filters were removed and tested using polymerase chain-reaction techniques to detect the presence of select pathogens, a labor-intensive process. In 2001 the system was tested with live microbes inside a sealed chamber at Dugway Proving Ground in Utah. It was tested for indoor and outdoor monitoring at the Salt Lake City Winter Olympics in 2002. The first positive incident was reported on October 9, 2003, in Houston, when the city's Department of Health and Human Services detected low levels of tularemia-causing bacterium for three days, though no human cases of the disease were reported. For more information, see Global Security, "Biowatch" and "Biological Aerosol Sentry and Information System (BASIS)." See also Roos, "Signs of Tularemia Agent Detected in Houston Air."

37 Despite numerous technical problems, the program continued into the second decade of the twenty-first century, coming to the public's attention again in June 2012, when a former Arizona governor and U.S. diplomat, Raul Castro, was detained at a checkpoint near the U.S.-Mexico border for more than an hour in extreme heat because he set off a radiation sensor. It turned out that his pacemaker and a medical procedure he had received the day before triggered the alarm. He was traveling with his wife and a friend from Nogales to Tucson for his ninety-sixth birthday party when the car triggered a radiation sensor. Daniel Gonzalez, "Agents Stir Outcry by Detaining Former Arizona Governor Raul Castro, 96," *Arizona Republic*, July 4, 2012, accessed June 5, 2015, http://www.azcentral.com/news/articles/2012/07/03/20120703agents-stir-outcry-by-detaining-former-arizona-governor-castro.html.

38 Shea, "The National Biodefense Analysis and Countermeasures Center."

39 Leitenberg et al., "Biodefense Crossing the Line"; Ember, "Testing the Limits."

40 Leitenberg, *Assessing the Biological Weapons and Bioterrorism Threat*; Tucker, "Biological Threat Assessment."

41 Nelson Hernandez, "Protesters Decry Fort Detrick Expansion," *Washington Post*, June 6, 2005. See also Federation of American Scientists, "The National Biodefense Analysis and Countermeasures Center."

42 Oswald, "Synthetic Biology Industry Poses Security Challenges, Experts Say."

43 Jo Warrick, "The Secretive Fight against Bioterror," *Washington Post*, July 30, 2006, accessed March 14, 2016, https://www.washingtonpost.com/archive

/politics/2006/07/30/the-secretive-fight-against-bioterror-span-classbank
headthe-government-is-building-a-highly-classified-facility-to-research
-biological-weapons-but-its-closed-door-approach-has-raised-concerns-span
/17933fac-8e79-4692-b672-c3096411ab40/?resType=accessibility.

44 For an overview, see Grotton, "Project BioShield."

45 The comment was made by a Boston University law professor, Kevin Outterson, and quoted in Gorenstein, "BARDA."

46 Andrew Bridges, "An Agency, Quietly, Would Spur Vaccines: Federal Bill Seeks to Shield Bureau from Public Review," *Boston Globe*, December 4, 2005, accessed July 23, 2015, http://www.boston.com/news/nation/articles/2005/12/04/an _agency_quietly_would_spur_vaccines/.

47 "Senate Panel Backs Special Vaccine Agency," *USA Today*, December 2, 2005, accessed July 23, 2015, http://usatoday30.usatoday.com/news/washington/2005 -12-02-vaccine-agency_x.htm.

48 Jim Drinkard, "Drugmakers Go Furthest to Sway Congress," *USA Today*, April 25, 2005, accessed July 23, 2015, http://usatoday30.usatoday.com/news /health/2005-04-25-drug-lobby-cover_x.htm.

49 Burr, "Senate Passes Burr's Bipartisan Biodefense and Pandemic Preparedness Legislation," emphasis added.

50 U.S. Congress, Pandemic and All-Hazards Preparedness Act.

51 Hayden, "Pentagon Rethinks Bioterror Effort."

52 In *Life as Surplus* Melinda Cooper writes that the concept of *emergence* in biowarfare and disaster management is tied to the term's currency in economic discourse. Venture capital redefines *productivity* as the capacity to take advantage of unforeseen or unforeseeable situations. In this context we find what Cooper calls the professional speculator, who is able to sense a trend before it takes hold and to mobilize investors' sentiments—whether confidence, euphoria, or panic—in anticipation of an event that has not yet materialized. Biotechnology and information technology, two sectors of the economy where venture capital has been concentrated since the Reagan-era deregulation of financial institutions, offer promises of life-enhancing soon-to-be-realized products. Talk of emergent threats and emergent diseases provokes talk of emergent investment opportunities. At a time of feverishly nomadic speculation among venture capitalists, it matters less whether a company's product turns a profit than if your promise attracts shareholders. The speculator moves on before the losses set in, with the insurance policy of either betting on losses or on government bailouts. Cooper argues that Bush's war on bioterrorism was a political response to the downturn of the dot-com economy in 2000. Large-scale funding sources such as Project BioShield could bail out a flagging biotech sector, which by the end of the 1990s had yet to turn a profit. The Human Genome Project had not successfully turned its DNA sequencing into valuable and profitable medical products, and investors felt burned. Biodefense could possibly rescue a faltering biotech industry. Contrasted to the hope evident in Clinton's embrace of innovation

that generated short-lived promises, the Bush era emphasized the indefinite dangers of the Global War on Terror, in which permanent warfare could become a renewed driving force behind U.S. economic growth. That was the hope, at least. The Great Recession of 2007–9, resulting from the trading of toxic derivatives on subprime mortgages and the bursting of an $8 trillion housing bubble, proved that hope to be misplaced.

53 Rajan, *Biocapital.*

54 Hayden, "Biodefense since 9/11."

55 Cohen, "Reinventing Project BioShield," 1216, quoting National Biodefense Science Board, "Where Are the Countermeasures?"

56 Cohen, "Reinventing Project BioShield," 1216.

57 U.S. Centers for Disease Control and Prevention, "The 2009 H1N1 Pandemic."

58 Dana Priest and Anne Hull, "Soldiers Face Neglect, Frustration at Army's Top Medical Facility," *Washington Post*, February 18, 2007, accessed July 15, 2015, http://www.washingtonpost.com/wp-dyn/content/article/2007/02/17/AR2007021701172.html. See also Richard A. Oppel Jr. and Michael D. Shear, "Severe Report Finds V.A. Hid Waiting Lists at Hospitals," *New York Times*, May 28, 2014, accessed May 30, 2014, http://www.nytimes.com/2014/05/29/us/va-report-confirms-improper-waiting-lists-at-phoenix-center.html.

59 U.S. Congress, "Is Military Research Hazardous to Veterans' Health?"

60 Jim Carlton, "Of Microbes and Mock Attacks: Years Ago, the Military Sprayed Germs on U.S. Cities," *Wall Street Journal*, October 22, 2001, accessed July 15, 2015, http://www.wsj.com/articles/SB1003703226697496080.

61 Washington, *Medical Apartheid*, 359–65.

62 Washington, *Medical Apartheid*, 360.

63 The CIA conducted secret experiments through the MK-ULTRA, nicknamed the CIA's mind-control program because it focused on research and development of drugs and other techniques that could be used to alter brain function, chief among them LSD, hypnosis, and electroshock. The ultrasecret program was ordered by CIA director Allen Dulles and headed by Sidney Gottlieb to develop drugs to be used against Cold War opponents during interrogations. A congressional committee chaired by Senator Frank Church III, an Idaho Democrat, and a presidential commission headed by John D. Rockefeller IV, a Democrat from West Virginia, investigated the program in 1975 in the wake of investigative reporting that uncovered evidence of illegal activities carried out since the early 1950s by the CIA. Richard Helms, CIA director, had destroyed many of the files in 1973, which obstructed the committee's investigation. MK-ULTRA was carried out by 185 private researchers through subcontracts with some eighty unwitting organizations, including universities, prisons, hospitals, and pharmaceutical companies. Based on the recommendations of the Church committee, President Gerald Ford issued an Executive Order in 1976 that prohibited experimentation on human subjects, except with informed consent in writing and witnessed by a disinterested party. In 1977 a Freedom of Information Act

request brought to light twenty thousand more documents about the program, sparking Senate hearings that uncovered the extensive testing and experimentation of the program that had resulted in at least one death. Dr. Frank Olson, a U.S. Army biochemist and biological weapons researcher, had been administered LSD against his knowledge and consent in November 1953. A week later he threw himself out of the window from his thirteenth-floor hotel room. Olson had quit his position as acting chief of the Special Operations Division at Fort Detrick a few days before his death. His family insisted that he resigned because of a deep moral crisis about the government's biological weapons research. See U.S. Congress, *Final Report of the Select Committee to Study Governmental Operations with Respect to Intelligence Activities, Foreign and Military Intelligence*. For more on Olson's death, see Frank Olson Legacy Project, "Family Statement on the Murder of Frank Olson."

64 Bill Richards, "Report Suggests CIA Involvement in Fla. Illness," *Washington Post*, December 17, 1979.

65 U.S. Congress, "Is Military Research Hazardous to Veterans' Health?," 47.

66 U.S. Congress, "Is Military Research Hazardous to Veterans' Health?," 36.

67 Quoted in Washington, *Medical Apartheid*, 370.

68 As of June 2015, the CDC reported that no cases of H5 bird flu virus in humans had been detected in the United States. However, between December 2014 and mid-June 2015 detections in birds were reported in twenty-one states (fifteen states with outbreaks in domestic poultry or captive birds and six with H5 detections only in wild birds). See U.S. Centers for Disease Control and Prevention, "H5 Viruses in the United States."

69 Schwartz, "The Tamiflu Tug of War." See also Schwartz, "Rumsfeld's Growing Stake in Tamiflu."

70 Federation of American Scientists, "Harkin Amendment for Avian Flu Funding Passes!"

EPILOGUE

1 Stewart, "Worlding."

2 This dilemma is discussed in Fassin, *Humanitarian Reason*, 225–27.

3 For more on the history of the Women's International League for Peace and Freedom, see Foster, *Women for All Seasons*; Schott, *Reconstructing Women's Thoughts*.

4 Blackwell, *No Peace without Freedom*.

5 Swerdlow, *Women Strike for Peace*.

6 The Papers of the Women's Encampment for a Future of Peace and Justice are housed in the Schlesinger Library at Radcliffe College, Cambridge, Massachusetts. The Women's Video Project recorded many of the protests of the camp. These can be found along with recorded oral histories at the Peace Encampment

Herstory Project, http://peacecampherstory.blogspot.com/2014/10/blog-post _5.html.

7   IVAW board director Sara Beining enlisted at seventeen to become an intelligence analyst in 2004. She was stationed at Fort Hood before being deployed to Iraq from December 2005 through November 2006. She went AWOL two times, once in January 2007, a few months after she spontaneously joined an IVAW protest march, and again in 2013. Kelly Dougherty was the secretary of the board. She joined the Colorado Army National Guard in 1996 at seventeen and enlisted as a medic but was deployed as Military Police, once in 1999–2000 to Croatia and then to Kuwait and Iraq in 2003–4. She recalled that she "[drove] around endlessly, antagonized and harassed Iraqis, and secured corporate profits for [private contractor] KBR." She attended the 2004 convention when the IVAW was formed and went on to be its executive director from 2006 to 2009. See the women's full biographies at the IVAW website, http://www.ivaw.org /about/board.

8   See Hedges, "The Last Days of Tomas Young"; Spiro and Donahue, *Body of War*.

9   My reference here is to the antebellum Negro spiritual "Down by the Riverside," whose lyrics incorporate Isaiah 2:4. The song was revived in the 1960s as a protest song during the Vietnam War.

BIBLIOGRAPHY

Abraham, Laurie Kaye. *Mama Might Be Better Off Dead: The Failure of Health Care in Urban America.* Chicago: University of Chicago Press, 1993.

ACLU. "ACLU Releases Files on Civilian Casualties in Afghanistan and Iraq." April 12, 2007. Accessed July 1, 2015. https://www.aclu.org/news/aclu-releases -files-civilian-casualties-afghanistan-and-iraq?redirect=cpredirect/29316.

Adams, Vincanne. *Markets of Sorrow, Labors of Faith: New Orleans in the Wake of Katrina.* Durham, N.C.: Duke University Press, 2013.

Adams, Vincanne, Michelle Murphy, and Adele E. Clarke. "Anticipation: Technoscience, Life, Affect, Temporality." *Subjectivity* 28 (2009): 246–65.

Adee, Sally. "Winner: The Revolution Will Be Prosthetized." *IEEE Spectrum*, January 1, 2009. Accessed July 17, 2014. http://spectrum.ieee.org/robotics/medical -robots/winner-the-revolution-will-be-prosthetized.

AFIRM. "Our Science for Their Healing." Annual Report, 2011.

Ahuja, Neel. *Bioinsecurities: Disease Interventions, Empire, and the Government of Species.* Durham, N.C.: Duke University Press, 2016.

Alexander, Caroline. "Rivaling Nature: The War in Iraq Has Increased Demand for Limb and Facial Plastic Surgeons." *Smithsonian Magazine*, February 2007. Accessed July 31, 2014. http://www.smithsonianmag.com/history/rivaling -nature-145879738/?no-ist.

Ali, Mohamed, John Blacker, and Gareth Jones. "Annual Mortality Rates and Excess Deaths of Children under Five in Iraq, 1991–98." *Population Studies* 57.2 (2003): 217–26.

Anderson, Chelsea. "Marine Wounded Warrior Offered Bittersweet Opportunity." *Marines Blog: The Official Blog of the United States Marine Corps*, April 9, 2013. Accessed April 12, 2014. https://www.dvidshub.net/news/104892/marine -wounded-warrior-offered-bittersweet-opportunity.

Anderson, Warwick. *Colonial Pathologies: American Tropical Medicine, Race, and Hygiene in the Philippines.* Durham, N.C.: Duke University Press, 2006.

Annas, George J. "Hunger Strikes at Guantanamo: Medical Ethics and Human Rights in a 'Legal Black Hole.'" *New England Journal of Medicine* 355 (2006): 1377–82.

Appadurai, Arjun. "Disjunction and Difference in the Global Cultural Economy." *Public Culture* 2.20 (1990): 295–310.

Arms Control Association. *Biological Weapons Convention*, March 26, 1975. Accessed May 4, 2014. https://www.armscontrol.org/treaties/biological-weapons -convention.

Asch, Adrienne. "Appearance-Altering Surgery, Children's Sense of Self, and Parental Love." In *Surgically Shaping Children: Technology, Ethics, and the Pursuit of Normality*, ed. Erik Parens, 227–52. Baltimore: Johns Hopkins University Press, 2006.

Bacher, Jamie M., Brian D. Reiss, and Andrew D. Ellington. "Anticipatory Evolution and DNA Shuffling." *Genome Biology* 3.8 (2002): 1021–25.

Baker, S. P., B. O'Neill, W. Haddon Jr., and W. B. Long. "The Injury Severity Score: A Method for Describing Patients with Multiple Injuries and Evaluating Emergency Care." *Journal of Trauma* 14 (1974): 187–96.

Baptist Medical Center, Wake Forest. "Institute for Regenerative Medicine to Lead National Effort to Aid Wounded Warriors." September 27, 2013. Accessed May 4, 2014. http://www.wakehealth.edu/News-Releases/2013/Institute_for _Regenerative_Medicine_to_Lead_National_Effort_to_Aid_Wounded_ Warriors.htm.

———. "Scientists Successfully Grow Animal Penile Erectile Tissue in Lab." Press Release. November 4, 2009. Accessed May 1, 2014. http://www.newswise.com /articles/view/558223/?sc=dwhr;xy=5028683.

Bashford, Alison. *Imperial Hygiene: A Critical History of Colonialism, Nationalism, and Public Health*. New York: Palgrave Macmillan, 2004.

———. *Medicine at the Borders: Disease, Globalization, and Security: 1850 to the Present*. New York: Palgrave Macmillan, 2006.

Bashford, Alison, and Claire Hooker, eds. *Contagion: Historical and Cultural Studies*. New York: Routledge, 2001.

Baudrillard, Jean. *The Transparency of Evil*. Trans. James Benedict. London: Verso, 1993.

Beard, Jonathan. "DARPA's Bio-Revolution: An Array of Programs Aim to Improve the Safety, Health, and Well-Being of the Military and Civilians Alike." In *DARPA: 50 Years of Bridging the Gap*, DARPA, April 2008, 155–60. Accessed March 13, 2017. http://cdn.mashreghnews.ir/old/files/fa/news/1390/10/26 /127214_872.pdf.

Becker, Gary. "Health as Human Capital: Synthesis and Extensions." *Oxford Economic Papers* 59.3 (2007): 379–410.

Belfiore, Michael. *The Department of Mad Scientists: How DARPA Is Remaking Our World, from the Internet to Artificial Limbs*. Washington, D.C.: Smithsonian, 2009.

Bell, Colleen. "Hybrid Warfare and Its Metaphors." *Humanity* 3.2 (2012): 225–47.

———. "War and the Allegory of Medical Intervention." *International Political Sociology* 6.3 (2012): 325–28.

Benanav, Aaron, and John Clegg. "Misery and Debt: On the Logic and History of Surplus Populations and Surplus Capital." *Endnotes*, no. 2 (2010). https://end notes.org.uk/articles/1.

Benard, Cheryl, Seth G. Jones, Olga Oliker, Chatryn Quantic Thurston, Brooke K. Stearns, and Kristen Cordell. *Women and Nation-Building*. Santa Monica, Calif.: RAND, 2008.

Bender, Leonard. *Prosthesis and Rehabilitation after Arm Amputation*. Springfield, Ill.: Charles C. Thomas, 1974.

Benjamin, Ruha. *People's Science: Bodies and Rights on the Stem Cell Frontier*. Palo Alto: Stanford University Press, 2013.

Bennett, Jane. *Vibrant Matter: A Political Ecology of Things*. Durham, N.C.: Duke University Press, 2010.

Berlant, Lauren. *Cruel Optimism*. Durham, N.C.: Duke University Press, 2011.

———. "On Citizenship and Optimism." Interview by David Seitz. *Society and Space: An Interdisciplinary Journal*, March 22, 2013. Accessed January 1, 2014. http://societyandspace.org/2013/03/22/on-citizenship-and-optimism/.

Bilmes, Linda. "Soldiers Returning from Iraq and Afghanistan: The Long-Term Costs of Providing Veterans Medical Care and Disability Benefits." Faculty Research Working Papers Series. John F. Kennedy School of Government, Harvard University, January 2007. Accessed July 1, 2015. http://papers.ssrn.com/sol3/papers.cfm?abstract_id=939657.

Biological Technologies Office. DARPA. Accessed June 3, 2014. http://www.darpa.mil/about-us/offices/bto.

Biomechatronics Group. "About." Accessed June 20, 2014. http://biomech.media.mit.edu/#/about/.

"The Bionic Man Who Builds Bionic People." *Discover*, January 25, 2011, 1. Accessed June 24, 2014. http://discovermagazine.com/2010/nov/25-bionic-man-who-builds-people.

Blackwell, Joyce. *No Peace without Freedom: Race and the Women's International League for Peace and Freedom, 1915–1975*. Carbondale: Southern Illinois University Press, 2004.

Blough, David K., Sharon Hubbard, Lynne V. McFarland, Douglas C. Smith, Jeffrey M. Gambel, and Gayle E. Reibe. "Prosthetic Cost Projections for Servicemembers with Major Limb Loss from Vietnam and OIF/OEF." *Journal of Rehabilitation Research and Development* 47.4 (2010): 387–402.

Bowlby, John. *Attachment and Loss*. Vol. 1: *Attachment*. 2nd ed. New York: Basic Books, 1982.

———. *Attachment and Loss*. Vol. 3: *Loss: Sadness and Depression*. London: Hogarth, 1980.

———. "Grief and Mourning in Infancy and Early Childhood." *Psychiatric Study of the Child* 15 (1960): 9–52.

———. *Maternal Care and Mental Health*. Report. Geneva: World Health Organization, 1952.

———. "The Nature of the Child's Tie to His Mother." *International Journal of Psycho-Analysis* 39 (1958): 350–73.

———. *Separation Anxiety and Anger*. 1959; New York: Basic Books, 1976.

Burr, Richard. "Senate Passes Burr's Bipartisan Biodefense and Pandemic Preparedness Legislation." Press release. December 5, 2006. Accessed August 20, 2014.
http://www.burr.senate.gov/press/releases/senate-passes-burrs-bipartisan
-biodefense-and-pandemic-preparedness-legislation.

Bush, George W. Executive Order 13435: "Expanding Approved Stem Cell Lines in Ethically Responsible Ways." June 20, 2007. Accessed May 1, 2014. https://george
wbush-whitehouse.archives.gov/news/releases/2007/06/20070620-6.html.

———. "Landon Lecture." January 23, 2006. Kansas State University, Media Relations. Accessed June 9, 2015. http://www.k-state.edu/media/newsreleases
/landonlect/bushtext106.html.

———. "The National Security Strategy of the United States of America." The
White House. September 17, 2002. Accessed July 2, 2015. http://www
.informationclearinghouse.info/article2320.htm.

———. "President Discusses Stem Cell Research." The White House. August 9,
2001. Accessed May 4, 2014. https://georgewbush-whitehouse.archives.gov
/news/releases/2001/08/20010809-2.html.

———. "State of the Union Address." January 29, 2002. *American Rhetoric Online
Speech Bank.* Accessed January 7, 2010. http://www.americanrhetoric.com
/speeches/stateoftheunion2002.htm.

———. "State of the Union Address." January 28, 2003. *Washington Post.* Accessed
June 9, 2015. http://www.washingtonpost.com/wp-srv/onpolitics/transcripts
/bushtext_012803.html.

Bush, Vannevar. *Science, the Endless Frontier: A Report to the President on a Program
for Postwar Scientific Research.* Washington, D.C.: U.S. Government Printing
Office, 1945.

Business Innovation Factory. "Hugh Herr at BIF-2." Accessed April 16, 2014. http://
www.businessinnovationfactory.com/summit/story/hugh-herr-bif-2.

———. "Hugh Herr: Director, Biomechatronics, MIT Media Lab." Accessed April 16,
2014. http://www.businessinnovationfactory.com/iss/innovators/hugh-herr.

Cabot, Tyler. "Whatever Happened to Stem Cells?" *Esquire*, March 18, 2013. Accessed May 7, 2014. http://www.esquire.com/features/stem-cells-research
-politics-0413.

Caidin, Martin. *Cyborg.* New York: Del Rey, 1984.

Cartwright, Lisa, and Brian Goldfarb. "On the Subject of Neural and Sensory Pros-
theses." In *The Prosthetic Impulse: From a Posthuman Present to a Biocultural
Future*, ed. Marquard Smith and Joanna Morra, 125–54. Cambridge, Mass.:
MIT Press, 2006.

Chen, Kuan-Hsing, and David Morley, eds. *Stuart Hall: Critical Dialogues in Cultural
Studies.* New York: Routledge, 1996.

Chen, Kuo-Liang, Daniel Eberli, James J. Yoo, and Anthony Atala. "Bioengineered
Corporal Tissue for Structural and Functional Restoration of the Penis."
Proceedings of the National Academy of Science 107.8 (2010): 3346–50. Published
online on November 13, 2009.

Clarke, Adele E., Janet K. Shim, Laura Mamo, Jennifer Ruth Fosket, and Jennifer R. Fishman. "Biomedicalization: Technoscientific Transformations of Health, Illness, and U.S. Biomedicine." In *Biomedicalization: Technoscience, Health, and Illness in the U.S.*, ed. Adele E. Clarke et al., 47–87. Durham, N.C.: Duke University Press, 2010.

Cohen, Jon. "Reinventing Project BioShield." *Science* 2 (September 2011): 1216–18.

Conover, Chris. "Bullets vs. Band-Aids: Is Health Spending Crowding Out Defense?" *Forbes*, February 12, 2013. Accessed June 15, 2015. http://www.forbes.com/sites/chrisconover/2013/02/12/bullets-vs-band-aids-is-health-spending-crowding-out-defense/.

Cooper, Melinda. *Life as Surplus: Biotechnology and Capitalism in the Neoliberal Era.* Minneapolis: University of Minnesota Press, 2008.

Crawford, Cassandra S. *Phantom Limb: Amputation, Embodiment, and Prosthetic Technology.* New York: New York University Press, 2014.

Crawford, Neta C. "Civilian Death and Injury in Afghanistan, 2001–2011." *Costs of War*. Watson Institute for International and Public Affairs, Brown University. September 2011. Accessed January 22, 2014. http://watson.brown.edu/costsofwar/files/cow/imce/papers/2011/Civilian%20Death%20and%20Injury%20in%20Afghanistan,%202001-2011.pdf.

Crosby, Sondra J., Caroline M. Apovian, and Michael A. Grodin. "Hunger Strikes, Force-Feeding and Physicians' Responsibilities." *Journal of the American Medical Association* 298.5 (2007): 563–66.

Dando, Malcolm. *Bioterror and Biowarfare: A Beginner's Guide.* Oxford: Oneworld, 2006.

DARPA. "DARPA Launches Biological Technologies Office." Press release. April 1, 2014. Accessed February 26, 2017. http://www.darpa.mil/news-events/2014-04-01.

———. "From Idea to Market in Eight Years: DARPA-Funded DEKA Arm System Earns FDA Approval." May 9, 2014. Accessed February 26, 2017. http://www.darpa.mil/news-events/2014-05-09.

"Deans Protest Sham Vaccination Program in Pakistan." *Newsletter of the Columbia University Mailman School of Public Health*, January 9, 2013. Accessed June 15, 2015. http://www.mailman.columbia.edu/news/deans-protest-sham-vaccination-program-pakistan.

Dentzer, Susan. "Prosthetic Sculptures Duplicate Faces of Wounded U.S. Soldiers." *PBS NewsHour*, October 12, 2006. Accessed April 3, 2014. http://www.pbs.org/newshour/bb/health-july-dec06-hanson_10-11/.

DePalma, Ralph G., David G. Burris, Howard R. Champion, and Michael J. Hodgson. "Blast Injuries." *New England Journal of Medicine* 352.13 (2005): 1335–42.

Dewachi, Omar, Mac Skelton, Vinh-Kim Nguyen, Fouad M. Fouad, Ghassan Abu Sitta, Zeina Maasri, and Rita Giacaman. "Changing Therapeutic Geographies of the Iraq and Syrian Wars." *Lancet* 383 (February 1, 2014): 449–57. Accessed June 15, 2015. http://www.thelancet.com/journals/lancet/article/PIIS0140-6736(13)62299-0/fulltext.

Donaldson, Ross I., Patrick Shanovich, Pranav Shetty, Emma Clark, Sharaf Aziz, Melinda Morton, Tariq Hasoon, and Gerald Evans. "A Survey of National Physicians Working in an Active Conflict Zone: The Challenges of Emergency Medical Care in Iraq." *Prehospital and Disaster Medicine* 27 (2012): 153–61.

Donoghue, John P. "Connecting Cortex to Machines: Recent Advances in Brain Interfaces." *Nature Neuroscience* 5 (2002): 1085–88.

Drummond, Katie. "World's Most Wired War Healer: Joachim Kohn." *Wired*, September 24, 2012. Accessed April 2, 2014. http://www.wired.com/2012/09 /worlds-most-wired-joachim-kohn/.

Drury, Bob. *Signature Wound: Hidden Bombs, Heroic Soldiers, and the Shocking Secret of the Afghanistan War*. Emmaus, Pa.: Rodale/Men's Health Books, 2011.

Eastman, Guy, and Fenella McGerty. "Analysis: U.S. No Longer Spends More on Defense than Next 10 Biggest Countries Combined." *IHS Jane's 360*, June 25, 2014. Accessed June 15, 2015. http://www.janes.com/article/40083/analysis-us -no-longer-spends-more-on-defense-than-next-10-biggest-countries-combined.

Edwards, M. J., M. Lustik, M. R. Eichelberger, E. Elster, K. Azarow, and C. Coppola. "Blast Injury in Children: An Analysis from Afghanistan and Iraq, 2002–2010." *Journal of Trauma and Acute Care Surgery* 73.5 (2012): 1278–83.

Eisenhower, Dwight D. "Farewell Address to the Nation." Dwight D. Eisenhower Presidential Archives. January 17, 1961. Accessed February 26, 2017. https:// www.eisenhower.archives.gov/research/online_documents/farewell_address /1961_01_17_Press_Release.pdf.

Elbe, Stefan. "Bodies as Battlefields: Toward a Medicalization of Insecurity." *International Political Sociology* 6.3 (2012): 320–22.

Ember, Lois R. "Testing the Limits." *Chemical and Engineering News*, August 15, 2005, 26–32. Accessed April 2, 2014. http://pubs.acs.org/cen/government/83 /8333gov1.html.

Enloe, Cynthia. "How Do They Militarize a Can of Soup?" In *Maneuvers: The International Politics of Militarizing Women's Lives*, 1–14. Berkeley: University of California Press, 2000.

Fanon, Frantz. *A Dying Colonialism*. Trans. Haakon Chevalier. New York: Grove Weidenfeld, 1965.

Farmer, Paul. *Infections and Inequalities: The Modern Plagues*. Berkeley: University of California Press, 2001.

———. *Pathologies of Power: Health, Human Rights, and the New War on the Poor*. Berkeley: University of California Press, 2004.

Fassin, Didier. *Humanitarian Reason: A Moral History of the Present*. Berkeley: University of California Press, 2012.

Fauci, Anthony, and Francis S. Collins. "Benefits and Risks of Influenza Research: Lessons Learned." *Science* 336 (June 22, 2012): 1522–23.

FBI. "Amerithrax or Anthrax Investigation." Accessed April 25, 2014. http://www .fbi.gov/about-us/history/famous-cases/anthrax-amerithrax/amerithrax -investigation.

Federation of American Scientists. "Harkin Amendment for Avian Flu Funding Passes!" April 5, 2006. Accessed February 26, 2017. https://fas.org/blogs/security/2006/04/harkin_amendment_for_avian_flu/.

———. "The National Biodefense Analysis and Countermeasures Center." Accessed February 26, 2017. https://fas.org/biosecurity/resource/nbacc.htm.

Fischer, Hannah. "A Guide to U.S. Military Casualty Statistics: Operation New Dawn, Operation Iraqi Freedom, and Operation Enduring Freedom." *Congressional Research Service*, February 19, 2014. Accessed June 30, 2014. http://fas.org/sgp/crs/natsec/RS22452.pdf.

FitzGerald, Mary C. *Marshal Ogarkov on Modern War: 1977–1985.* Professional Paper 443.10. Alexandria, Va.: Center for Naval Analyses, Hudson Institute, 1986.

Forte, Maximillian C. "The Human Terrain System and Anthropology: A Review of Ongoing Debates." *Public Anthropology* 113.1 (2011): 149–53.

Foster, Catherine. *Women for All Seasons: The Story of the Women's International League for Peace and Freedom.* Athens: University of Georgia Press, 1989.

Foucault, Michel. *The Birth of the Clinic: An Archaeology of Medical Perception.* Trans. A. M. Sheridan. New York: Vintage, 1994.

———. *The History of Sexuality.* Vol. 1: *An Introduction.* Trans. Robert Hurley. New York: Vintage, 1990.

———. *Lectures at the Collège de France, 1975–1976.* Vol. 3: *Society Must Be Defended.* Ed. Mauro Bertani and Alessandro Fontana. Trans. David Macey. New York: Palgrave Macmillan, 2003.

———. *Lectures at the Collège de France, 1977–1978.* Vol. 4: *Security, Territory, Population.* Ed. Michel Senellart, François Ewald, and Alessandro Fontana. Trans. Graham Burchell. New York: Palgrave Macmillan, 2009.

———. *Lectures at the Collège de France, 1978–1979.* Vol. 5: *The Birth of Biopolitics.* Ed. Michel Senellart. Trans. Graham Burchell. New York: Palgrave Macmillan, 2008.

———. "Technologies of the Self." In *The Essential Foucault*, ed. Paul Rabinow and Nikolas Rose, 145–69. New York: New Press, 2003.

Frank Olson Legacy Project. "Family Statement on the Murder of Frank Olson." August 8, 2002. Accessed January 3, 2016. http://www.frankolsonproject.org/Statements/FamilyStatement2002.html.

Freud, Anna, and Dorothy Burlingham. *Infants without Families: The Case for and against Residential Nurseries.* New York: International University Press, 1944.

"The Future of Artificial Limbs." *The Week*, March 22, 2014. Accessed July 7, 2014. http://theweek.com/article/index/258459/the-future-of-artificial-limbs.

Garfield, Richard. "Civilian Mortality after the 2003 Invasion." *Lancet* 381 (March 16, 2013): 877–79.

Garland-Thomson, Rosemary. "Cultural Logic of Euthanasia: 'Sad Fancyings' in Herman Melville's 'Bartleby.'" *American Literature* 76.4 (2004): 777–806.

Garrett, Laurie. *Betrayal of Trust: The Collapse of Global Public Health.* New York: Hyperion, 2000.

Gawande, Atul. "Casualties of War—Military Care for the Wounded from Iraq and Afghanistan." *New England Journal of Medicine* 351 (December 9, 2004): 2471–75.

Geissler, Erhard, and John Ellis van Courtland Moon, eds. *Biological and Toxin Weapons: Research, Development and Use from the Middle Ages to 1945.* New York: Oxford University Press, 1999.

Gilbert, Emily, and Corey Ponder. "Between Tragedy and Farce: 9/11 Compensation and the Value of Life and Death." *Antipode* 46.2 (2014): 404–25.

Global Security. "Biological Aerosol Sentry and Information System (BASIS)." Accessed April 2, 2014. http://www.globalsecurity.org/security/systems/basis .htm.

———. "Biowatch." Accessed April 2, 2014. http://www.globalsecurity.org/security /systems/biowatch.htm.

Goodeve, Thyrza. "No Wound Ever Speaks for Itself." *Artforum*, January 1992, 70–74.

Gorenstein, Dan. "BARDA: The Venture Capital Firm Buried in the U.S. Government." *Marketplace*, October 30, 2014. Accessed July 21, 2015. http://www .marketplace.org/topics/health-care/barda-venture-capital-firm-buried-us -government.

Grewal, Inderpal. "Racial Sovereignty and 'Shooter' Violence." *Sikh Formations: Religion, Culture, Theory* 9.2 (2013): 1–12.

———. *Transnational America: Feminisms, Diasporas, Neoliberalisms.* Durham, N.C.: Duke University Press, 2005.

Grotton, Frank. "Project BioShield: Purposes and Authorities." *Congressional Research Service*, July 6, 2009. Accessed April 5, 2014. http://cironline.org/sites /default/files/legacy/files/July2009CRSbioshield.pdf.

"Growing Body Parts: Morley Safer Reports on the Amazing Science of Regenerative Medicine Growing Body Parts." *60 Minutes with Morley Safer*, December 13, 2009, updated July 25, 2010. Accessed April 11, 2014. http://www .cbsnews.com/news/growing-body-parts-21–07–2010/4/.

Guillemin, Jeanne. *American Anthrax: Fear, Crime, and the Investigation of the Nation's Deadliest Bioterrorist Attack.* New York: Macmillan/Henry Holt, 2011.

———. *Biological Weapons: From the Invention of State-Sponsored Programs to Contemporary Bioterrorism.* New York: Columbia University Press, 2006.

———. "Scientists and the History of Biological Weapons." *EMBO Reports* 7.S1 (July 2006): S45–S49. Accessed August 27, 2012. http://www.nature.com/embor /journal/v7/n1s/pdf/7400689.pdf.

Gunewardena, Nandini, and Mark Schuller, eds. *Capitalizing on Catastrophe: Neoliberal Strategies in Disaster Reconstruction.* New York: Rowman and Littlefield, 2008.

Hagopian, Amy, Abraham D. Flaxman, Tim K. Takaro, Sahar A. Esa Al Shatari, Julie Rajaratnam, Stan Becker, Alison Levin-Rector, Lindsay Galway, Berq J. Hadi Al-Yasseri, William M. Weiss, Christopher J. Murry, and Gilbert Burnhamd.

"Mortality in Iraq Associated with the 2003–2011 War and Occupation: Findings from a National Cluster Sample Survey by the University Collaborative Iraq Mortality Study." *PLOS Medicine* 10.10 (2013): 1–15. Accessed February 26, 2017. http://journals.plos.org/plosmedicine/article?id=10.1371/journal.pmed.1001533.

Hall, Stuart. "Cultural Studies and Its Theoretical Legacies." In *Stuart Hall: Critical Dialogues in Cultural Studies*, ed. Kuan-Hsing Chen and David Morley, 262–75. New York: Routledge, 1996.

Hanson Robotics. "About Hanson Robotics." Accessed June 29, 2014. http://www.hansonrobotics.com/about/.

Haraway, Donna J. "A Cyborg Manifesto: Science, Technology, and Socialist-Feminism in the Late Twentieth Century." In *Simians, Cyborgs, and Women: The Reinvention of Nature*, 149–81. London: Routledge, 1991.

———. "The Promises of Monsters: A Regenerative Politics for Inappropriate/d Others." In *Cultural Studies*, ed. Lawrence Grossberg, Cary Nelson, and Paula A. Treichler, 295–337. New York: Routledge, 1992.

———. *Staying with the Trouble: Making Kin in the Chthulucene*. Durham, N.C.: Duke University Press, 2016.

Hartman, Saidiya. *Lose Your Mother: A Journey along the Atlantic Slave Trade*. New York: Farrar, Straus and Giroux, 2008.

Harvey, E. Newton. "The Mechanism of Wounding by High Velocity Missiles." *Proceedings of the American Philosophical Society* 92.4 (1948): 294–304.

Harvey, E. Newton, J. Howard McMillen, Elmer G. Butler, and William O. Puckett. "Mechanism of Wounding." In *Wound Ballistics*, ed. James C. Beyer, 143–235. Washington, D.C.: U.S. Army Medical Department, 1962.

Haskell, Sally. "Post-deployment Health of OEF/OIF Women Veterans Who Use VA." Presentation to the National Training Summit on Women Veterans, July 16, 2011. Accessed February 26, 2017. https://www.va.gov/womenvet/docs/2011summit/2-Summit_HCbreakout_Haskell_FINAL.pdf.

Hastings, Michael. "The Runaway General." *Rolling Stone*, June 22, 2010. Accessed June 15, 2015. http://www.rollingstone.com/politics/news/the-runaway-general-20100622.

Hayden, Erika Check. "Biodefense since 9/11: The Price of Protection." *Nature* 477 (September 7, 2011): 150–52. Accessed July 20, 2012. http://www.nature.com/news/2011/110907/full/477150a.html.

———. "Pentagon Rethinks Bioterror Effort: Critics Say US $1.5 Billion Initiative Has Not Delivered Results." *Nature* 477 (September 21, 2011): 380–81. Accessed July 20, 2012. http://www.nature.com/news/2011/110921/full/477380a.html.

Hayles, N. Katherine. *How We Became Posthuman: Virtual Bodies in Cybernetics, Literature, and Informatics*. Chicago: University of Chicago Press, 1999.

Hedges, Chris. "The Last Days of Tomas Young." *Common Dreams*, November 17, 2014. Accessed August 20, 2015. http://www.commondreams.org/views/2014/11/17/last-days-tomas-young.

Hendren, John. "Balad Military Hospital Treats Soldiers, Insurgents." *All Things Considered*, NPR, March 23, 2006. Accessed April 4, 2014. http://www.npr.org /templates/story/story.php?storyId=5298089.

Henry J. Kaiser Foundation. "Snapshots: Health Care Spending in the United States and Selected OECD Countries." Report. April 12, 2011. Accessed July 10, 2012. http://kff.org/health-costs/issue-brief/snapshots-health-care-spending -in-the-united-states-selected-oecd-countries/.

Herr, Hugh. "The Double Amputee Who Designs Better Limbs." Interview by Terry Gross. *Fresh Air*, NPR, August 10, 2011. Accessed April 16, 2014. http://www .npr.org/2011/08/10/137552538/the-double-amputee-who-designs-better-limbs.

———. "The New Bionics That Let Us Run, Climb and Dance." TED Talk Vancouver, March 28, 2014. Accessed August 12, 2015. https://www.ted.com/talks/hugh _herr_the_new_bionics_that_let_us_run_climb_and_dance/transcript ?language=en.

Higgs, Robert. "Cleveland Clinic Doctors Perform First Almost-Total Face Transplant in the United States." *Cleveland.com*, December 16, 2008. Accessed August 14, 2014. http://blog.cleveland.com/medical/2008/12/cleveland_clinic _doctors_perfo.html.

Hipp, Van D., Jr. "How Military Medicine Is Leading the Way." *Rare: America's News Feed*, August 12, 2013. Accessed July 10, 2014. http://rare.us/story/how -military-medicine-is-leading-the-way/.

Hockenberry, John. *Moving Violations: War Zones, Wheelchairs and Declarations of Independence*. New York: Hyperion, 1995.

Hubbard, Ruth. "Science, Facts, and Feminism." *Hypatia* 3.1 (1988): 119–31.

International Committee of the Red Cross. "ICRC Survey: Our World—Views from the Field. Summary Report: Afghanistan, Colombia, Democratic Republic of the Congo, Georgia, Haiti, Lebanon, Liberia, and the Philippines." February 9, 2010. Accessed March 19, 2014. http://www.icrc.org/eng/resources/documents /publication/p1008.htm.

Iraq Body Count. "Iraqi Deaths from Violence, 2003–2011." January 2, 2012. Accessed June 22, 2015. https://www.iraqbodycount.org/analysis/numbers /2011/.

Iverson, Grant L. "Clinical and Methodological Challenges with Assessing Mild Traumatic Brain Injury in the Military." *Journal of Head Trauma Rehabilitation* 25.5 (2010): 313–19.

Ivey, Katherine M. "Improved Battlefield Triage and Transport May Raise Survival Rates for Severely Wounded Soldiers." *American College of Surgeons*, October 4, 2012. Accessed April 9, 2014. https://www.facs.org/media/press%20releases /cc2012/ivey.

Jabri, Vivienne. *War and the Transformation of Global Politics*. New York: Palgrave Macmillan, 2010.

Jain, Sarah. "The Prosthetic Imagination: Enabling and Disabling the Prosthesis Trope." *Science, Technology and Human Values* 24.1 (1999): 31–54.

Jayadev, Arjun. "Estimating Guard Labor." Working Paper 2. Political Economy Research Institute, University of Massachusetts at Amherst. February 2007. Accessed March 13, 2014. http://ideas.repec.org/p/mab/wpaper/7.html.

Jones, Ann. "Woman to Woman in Afghanistan." *Nation*, December 27, 2010. Accessed March 19, 2014. http://www.thenation.com/article/155623/woman -woman-afghanistan#.

Jurgenson, Nathan. "Against TED." *New Inquiry*, February 15, 2012. Accessed June 27, 2014. http://thenewinquiry.com/essays/against-ted/.

Kafer, Alison. *Feminist, Queer, Crip*. Bloomington: Indiana University Press, 2013.

Kagan, Donald, Gary Schmitt, and Thomas Donnelly. *Rebuilding America's Defenses: Strategies, Forces, and Resources for a New Century*. Report of Project for the New American Century, September 2000. Accessed December 20, 2016. https://web.archive.org/web/20130501130739/http://www.newamerican century.org/RebuildingAmericasDefenses.pdf.

Kaplan, Caren. "Precision Targets: GPS and the Militarization of U.S. Consumer Identity." *American Quarterly* 58.3 (2006): 693–714.

Kaplan, Caren, and Inderpal Grewal. "Transnational Practices and Interdisciplinary Feminist Scholarship: Refiguring Women's and Gender Studies." In *Women's Studies on Its Own: A Next Wave Reader in Institutional Change*, ed. Robyn Wiegman, 66–81. Durham, N.C.: Duke University Press, 2002.

Kaplan, Caren, Erik Loyer, and Ezra Claytan Daniels. "Precision Targets: GPS and the Militarization of Everyday Life." *Canadian Journal of Communication* 38.3 (2013): 397–420.

Kehoe, Karrie, and Craig Shaw. "Spreadsheets List Prices Paid for an Afghan Life, a Cow, and a Car." *Thomson Reuters Foundation News*, July 16, 2014. Accessed June 9, 2015. http://www.trust.org/item/20140716124054-a0sf5/.

Kenny, Katherine E. "The Biopolitics of Global Health: Life and Death in Neoliberal Time." *Journal of Sociology* 51.1 (2015): 9–27.

Khalili, Laleh. "Gendered Practices of Counterinsurgency." *Review of International Studies* 37.4 (2011): 1471–91.

———. "The New (and Old) Classics of Counterinsurgency." *Middle East Research and Information Project* 255 (2010). Accessed June 15, 2015. http://www.merip .org/mer/mer255/new-old-classics-counterinsurgency.

Kilcullen, David. *The Accidental Guerrilla: Fighting Small Wars in the Midst of a Big One*. Oxford: Oxford University Press, 2009.

———. "Twenty-Eight Articles: Fundamentals of Company-Level Counterinsurgency." *Small Wars Journal*, March 2006. Accessed March 19, 2014. http://www .smallwarsjournal.com/documents/28articles.pdf.

Kinsey, Alfred C., Wardell B. Pomeroy, and Clyde E. Martin. *Sexual Behavior in the Human Male*. 1948; Bloomington: Indiana University Press, 1998.

Klein, Naomi. *The Shock Doctrine: The Rise of Disaster Capitalism*. New York: Metropolitan Books, 2008.

Klime, Patricia. "Surgery, Treatments Can Restore Injured Troops' Sexual Function."

Military Times, December 29, 2014. Accessed April 24, 2015. http://www
.militarytimes.com/story/military/2014/12/29/wounded-troops-sexual
-function/20529563/.

Kristol, William, and Robert Kagan. "Toward a Neo-Reaganite Foreign Policy."
Foreign Affairs 75 (1996): 18–32.

Kuiken, Todd. "A Prosthetic Arm That 'Feels.'" *Global TED Talk*, October 2011. Accessed July 25, 2014. http://www.ted.com/talks/todd_kuiken_a_prosthetic
_arm_that_feels.

Kuniholm, Jonathan. "An Open-Source Approach to Better Prosthetics." Interview
by Dave Davies. *Fresh Air*, NPR, November 10, 2009. Accessed June 20, 2015.
http://www.npr.org/templates/story/story.php?storyId=120271945.

——. "We Have the Technology, Right?" TEDx Chapel Hill. *YouTube*, June 2,
2011. Accessed July 1, 2014. https://www.youtube.com/watch?v=7AWRSV
uN2ik.

Kurzman, Steven L. "Performing Able-Bodiedness: Amputees and Prosthetics in
America." PhD dissertation, University of California, Santa Cruz, 2003.

——. "Presence and Prosthesis: A Response to Nelson and Wright." *Cultural
Anthropology* 16.3 (2001): 374–87.

Lakoff, Andrew. "Two Regimes of Global Health." *Humanity: An International Journal of Human Rights, Humanitarianism, and Development* 1.1 (2010): 59–79.

Lane, Harlan. *The Mask of Benevolence: Disabling the Deaf Community*. New York:
Knopf, 1992.

Lawrence, Quil. "At Bagram, War's Tragedy Yields Medical Advances." *All Things
Considered*, NPR, December 29, 2010. Accessed April 3, 2014. http://www.npr
.org/2010/12/29/132437138/at-bagram-wars-tragedy-yields-medical-advances.

Lea, David. *Property Rights, Indigenous People and the Developing World: Issues from
Aboriginal Entitlement to Intellectual Ownership Rights*. Leiden: Martinus
Nijhoff, 2008.

League of Nations. "Protocol for the Prohibition of the Use in War of Asphyxiating,
Poisonous or Other Gases, and of Bacteriological Methods of Warfare." United
Nations Office for Disarmament Affairs. June 1925. Accessed August 27, 2012.
http://disarmament.un.org/treaties/t/1925/text.

Lehman, Cheryl. "Mechanisms of Injury in Wartime." *Rehabilitation Nursing* 33.5
(2008): 192–205.

Leick, Katya. "Stem Cells and Regenerative Medicine Help Kansans." KSNT, September 23, 2014. Accessed July 10, 2015. http://ksnt.com/2014/09/23/stem-cells
-and-regenerative-medicine-help-kansans/.

Leitenberg, Milton. *Assessing the Biological Weapons and Bioterrorism Threat*. Carlisle, Pa.: U.S. Army War College Press, 2005.

Leitenberg, Milton, James Leonard, and Richard Spertzel. "Biodefense Crossing the
Line." *Politics and the Life Sciences* 22 (2003): 2–3.

Levine, Phillipa. *Prostitution, Race, and Politics: Policing Venereal Disease in the British
Empire*. London: Routledge, 2003.

Levy, Barry S., and Victor W. Sidel. "Adverse Health Consequences of the Iraq War." *Lancet* 381 (March 16, 2013): 949–65.

Li, Tania. "To Make Live or Let Die? Rural Dispossession and the Protection of Surplus." *Antipode* 41.s1 (2009): 66–93.

Liachowitz, Claire H. *Disability as a Social Construct: Legislative Roots*. Philadelphia: University of Pennsylvania Press, 1988.

Lincoln, Bruce. *Holy Terrors: Thinking about Religion after September 11*. Chicago: University of Chicago Press, 2003.

Linker, Beth. *War's Waste: Rehabilitation in World War I America*. Chicago: University of Chicago Press, 2011.

Lorber, Deborah. "Better Care at Lower Cost: Is It Possible?" *The Commonwealth Fund*, November 21, 2013. Accessed January 15, 2014. http://www.common wealthfund.org/Publications/Health-Reform-and-You/Better-Care-at-Lower -Cost.aspx.

Love, Heather. *Feeling Backward: Loss and the Politics of Queer History*. Cambridge: Harvard University Press, 2007.

Lowe, Donald M. *The Body in Late-Capitalist USA*. Durham, N.C.: Duke University Press, 1995.

Lukes, H. M. "The Sovereignty of Subtraction: Hypo/Hyper Habilitation and the Cultural Politics of Amputation in America." *Social Text* 123.33 (2) (2015): 1–27.

Magnet, Shoshana. *When Biometrics Fail: Gender, Race, and the Technology of Identity*. Durham, N.C.: Duke University Press, 2011.

Manea, Octavian. "Reflections on the 'Counterinsurgency Decade': Small Wars Journal Interview." *Small Wars Journal*, September 1, 2013. Accessed April 9, 2014. http://smallwarsjournal.com/jrnl/art/reflections-on-the-counterinsurgency -decade-small-wars-journal-interview-with-general-david.

"Marine Captain Jon Kuniholm Speaks @ the 2008 DNC." *YouTube*, August 29, 2008. Accessed June 1, 2014. https://www.youtube.com/watch?v=g17yKwhwYvw.

Markets and Markets. "Medical Bionic Implant/Artificial Organs Market (Vision Bionics/Bionic Eye, Brain Bionics, Heart Bionics/Artificial Heart, Orthopedic Bionics and Ear Bionics): Trends and Global Forecasts to 2017." Report Number MD 1368. November 2012. Accessed April 20, 2013. http://www.markets andmarkets.com/Market-Reports/medical-bionic-implant-market-908.html.

Marmot, Michael, and Richard G. Wilkinson. *Social Determinants of Health*. Oxford: Oxford University Press, 2006.

Martin, Emily. *Flexible Bodies: The Role of Immunity in American Culture from the Days of Polio to the Age of AIDS*. Boston: Beacon, 1995.

Masco, Joseph. *The Theater of Operations: National Security Affect from the Cold War to the War on Terror*. Durham, N.C.: Duke University Press, 2014.

Mbembe, Achille. "Necropolitics." Trans. Libby Meintjes. *Public Culture* 15.1 (2003): 11–40.

McBride, Keally, and Annick T. R. Wibben. "The Gendering of Counterinsurgency in Afghanistan." *Humanity* 3.2 (2012): 199–215.

McCall, Ash. "Top 5 Army Medical Innovations—In Honor of National Patient Recognition Day." *U.S. Army Live, the Official Blog of the United States Army*, February 3, 2012. Accessed May 19, 2014. http://armylive.dodlive.mil/index .php/2012/02/top-5-army-medical-innovations-in-honor-of-national-patient -recognition-day/.

McNeill, J. R. *Mosquito Empires: Ecology and War in the Greater Caribbean, 1620– 1914.* Cambridge: Cambridge University Press, 2010.

Médecins sans Frontières / Doctors without Borders. "Special Report: The Ongoing Struggle to Access Healthcare in Afghanistan." February 24, 2014. Accessed February 26, 2014. http://www.doctorswithoutborders.org/article/special -report-ongoing-struggle-access-health-care-afghanistan.

Messinger, Seth. "Getting Past the Accident: Explosive Devices, Limb Loss, and Re- fashioning a Life in a Military Medical Center." *Medical Anthropology Quarterly* 24.3 (2010): 281–303.

———. "Medical Anthropology in a Military Treatment Facility." *Somatosphere*, February 8, 2011. Accessed June 23, 2015. http://somatosphere.net/2011/02 /medical-anthropology-in-military.html.

Metz, Steven, and James Kievit. "Strategy and the Revolution in Military Affairs: From Theory to Policy." Report submitted to the U.S. Army. June 27, 1995. Accessed July 28, 2015. http://www.au.af.mil/au/awc/awcgate/ssi/stratrma .pdf.

Michael, Markus. "Too Good to Be True? An Assessment of Health System Progress in Afghanistan, 2002–2012." *Medicine, Conflict and Survival* 29.4 (2013): 322–45.

"Mild Traumatic Brain Injury: Concussion." *Pocket Guide for Clinicians*, October 2010. Accessed April 11, 2014. http://www.publichealth.va.gov/docs/exposures /TBI-pocketcard.pdf.

Miles, Donna. "DARPA's Cutting-Edge Programs Revolutionize Prosthetics." U.S. Department of Defense, February 8, 2006. Accessed June 4, 2014. http://www .defense.gov/news/newsarticle.aspx?id=14914.

———. "Defense Agency Makes Big Advances in Prosthetics Research." U.S. De- partment of Defense Armed Forces Press Service, February 20, 2008. Accessed February 26, 2017. http://www.infozine.com/news/stories/op/storiesView /sid/27023/.

———. "Regenerative Medicine Shows Promise for Wounded Warriors." Armed Forces Press Service, February 25, 2010. Accessed February 26, 2017. http:// www.globalsecurity.org/military/library/news/2010/02/mil-100225-afps02 .htm.

Mitchell, David T., and Sharon L. Snyderman, eds. *The Body and Physical Differences: Discourses of Disability.* Ann Arbor: University of Michigan Press, 1997.

MIT Media Lab. "H2.0: New Minds, New Bodies, New Identities. Ushering in a New Era for Human Capability." Accessed July 4, 2014. http://h20.media.mit.edu /about.html.

Mitropoulos, Angela. *Contract and Contagion: From Biopolitics to Oikonomia.* New York: Minor Compositions, 2012.

Moisse, Katie. "The Lasting Fallout of Fake Vaccination Programs." *ABC News*, May 20, 2014. Accessed June 15, 2015. http://abcnews.go.com/Health/lasting -fallout-fake-vaccination-programs/story?id=23795483.

"Morbidity and Mortality among Families in Iraq." *Lancet* 371.9608 (2008): 177. Accessed March 18, 2014. http://www.thelancet.com/journals/lancet/article /PIIS0140673608601129/fulltext.

Mosley, Michael. "Miracles of War: How Front-Line Injuries Inform Modern Medicine." *Radio Times*, November 20, 2011.

Moturi, Edna K., Kimberly A. Porter, Steven G. F. Wassilak, Rudolf H. Tangermann, Ousmane M. Diop, Cara C. Burns, and Hamid Jafari. "Progress toward Polio Eradication—Worldwide, 2013–2014." U.S. Centers for Disease Control and Prevention, *Morbidity and Mortality Weekly Report*, May 30, 2014, 468–72. Accessed June 15, 2015. http://www.cdc.gov/mmwr/preview/mmwrhtml /mm6321a4.htm.

Mouffe, Chantal. *On the Political: Thinking in Action*. New York: Routledge, 2005.

Muñoz, José E. *Cruising Utopia: The Then and There of Queer Futurity*. Durham, N.C.: Duke University Press, 2009.

Murphy, Michelle. "Economization of Life: A Conversation with Leopold Lambert and Michelle Murphy: Archipelago Podcast Series." *The Funambulist*. Technoscience Research Unit, University of Toronto, November 22, 2014.

———. "Economization of Life: Calculative Infrastructures of Population and Economy." In *Relational Ecologies: Subjectivity, Sex, Nature and Architecture*, ed. Peg Rawes, 139–55. London: Routledge, 2013.

National Alliance to End Homelessness. "Vital Mission: Ending Homelessness among Veterans. 2008 Data and Policy Update." Accessed June 9, 2015. http://b.3cdn.net/naeh/c1c961005ocf6afbeo_fcm6iybab.pdf.

National Biodefense Science Board. "Where Are the Countermeasures? Protecting America's Health from CBRN Events." *Journal of Biosecurity and Bioterrorism* 8.2 (2010): 203–7.

Nguyen, Mimi Thi. *The Gift of Freedom: War, Debt, and Other Refugee Passages*. Durham, N.C.: Duke University Press, 2012.

Nordstrom, Carolyn. *Shadows of War: Violence, Power, and International Profiteering in the Twenty-First Century*. Berkeley: University of California Press, 2004.

North Carolina Biotechnology Center. "About Us." Accessed July 21, 2015. http:// www.ncbiotech.org/Connect.

Nye, David S., Jr. "Get Smart: Combining Hard and Soft Power." *Foreign Affairs* 88 (July/August 2009): 160–63.

Obama, Barack. Executive Order 13505: "Removing Barriers to Responsible Scientific Research Involving Human Stem Cells." March 9, 2009. Accessed December 20, 2016. https://www.whitehouse.gov/the-press-office/removing -barriers-responsible-scientific-research-involving-human-stem-cells.

O'Brien, Jeffrey M. "The Great Stem Cell Dilemma." *Fortune*, September 28, 2012. Accessed June 23, 2015. http://fortune.com/2012/09/28/the-great-stem-cell -dilemma/.

O'Connor, Erin. "'Fractions of Men:' Engendering Amputation in Victorian Culture." *Comparative Studies of Society and History* 39.4 (1997): 742–77.

Orr, Jackie. "The Militarization of Inner Space." *Critical Sociology* 30.2 (2004): 451–82.

Oswald, Rachel. "Synthetic Biology Industry Poses Security Challenges, Experts Say." *Global Security Newswire*, February 11, 2011. Accessed February 26, 2017. http://www.nti.org/gsn/article/synthetic-biology-industry-poses-security -challenges-experts-say/.

Ott, Katherine, David Serlin, and Stephen Mihm, eds. *Artificial Parts, Practical Lives: Modern Histories of Prosthesis.* New York: New York University Press, 2002.

Parens, Erik, and Adrienne Asch. "Disability Rights Critique of Prenatal Testing: Reflections and Recommendations." *Developmental Disabilities Research Reviews* 9.1 (2003): 40–47.

Park, Robert E. "Morale and the News." *American Journal of Sociology* 47.3 (1941): 360–77.

Peet, Judy. "Rutgers University Anchors U.S. Military Project in Regenerative Medicine." *New Jersey.com*, May 16, 2010. Accessed March 24, 2013. http://www .nj.com/news/index.ssf/2010/05/military_academic_consortium_m.html.

"The Pentagon's Bionic Arm: Pentagon Is Working to Develop a Life-Changing, High Tech Prosthetic Arm." *60 Minutes*, April 12, 2009. Accessed July 15, 2014. http://www.cbsnews.com/news/the-pentagons-bionic-arm/.

Perez-Rivas, Manuel. "Bush Vows to Rid the World of 'Evil-Doers.'" *CNN*, September 16, 2001. Accessed January 2, 2014. http://edition.cnn.com/2001/US/09 /16/gen.bush.terrorism/.

Physicians for Social Responsibility. "The Medical Consequences of the War in Iraq: Health Challenges beyond the Battlefield." September 29, 2007. Accessed May 12, 2014. http://www.psr-la.org/medical-consequences-war-in-iraq -conference/.

Pierce, Charles P. "Hugh Herr's New Parts: At MIT, Making 'Biohybrids,' or Prostheses That Blur the Line between Human and Device." *Esquire*, November 30, 2006. Accessed June 26, 2014. http://www.esquire.com/features/best-n -brightest-2006/ESQ1206HERRCONCRETE_186.

Pinchefsky, Carol. "Dmitry Itskov Wants to Live Forever. (He Wants You to Live Forever, Too.)" *Forbes*, June 18, 2013. Accessed August 15, 2014. http://www .forbes.com/sites/carolpinchefsky/2013/06/18/dmitry-itskov-wants-to-live -forever-he-wants-you-to-live-forever-too/.

Piore, Adam, and Scott Lewis. "How Pig Guts Became the Next Bright Hope for Regenerating Human Limbs." *Discover*, September 26, 2011. Accessed May 6, 2014. http://discovermagazine.com/2011/jul-aug/13-how-pig-guts-became -hope-regenerating-human-limbs.

Pottinger, Matt, Hali Jilani, and Claire Russo. "Half-Hearted: Trying to Win Afghanistan without Afghan Women." *Small Wars Journal*, February 18, 2010.

Accessed March 19, 2014. http://smallwarsjournal.com/jrnl/art/trying-to-win
-afghanistan-without-afghan-women.

Powell, Colin, with Tony Klotz. *It Worked for Me: In Life and Leadership*. New York:
Harper Perennial, 2012.

Priest, Dana, and William M. Arkin. *Top Secret America: The Rise of the New American Security State*. New York: Little, Brown, 2011.

Project for the New American Century. "Letter to Honorable William J. Clinton."
January 26, 1998. Accessed February 26, 2017. http://www.informationclearing
house.info/article5527.htm.

Public Intelligence. "Identity Dominance: The U.S. Military's Biometric War in
Afghanistan." April 21, 2014. Accessed June 15, 2015. http://publicintelligence
.net/identity-dominance/.

Rajan, Kaushik Sunder. *Biocapital: The Consumption of Postgenomic Life*. Durham,
N.C.: Duke University Press, 2006.

Rancière, Jacques. *Dissensus: On Politics and Aesthetics*. Trans. Steven Corcoran.
New York: Bloomsbury, 2015.

Rapp, Rayna. *Testing Women, Testing the Fetus: The Social Impact of Amniocentesis in
America*. New York: Routledge, 2000.

Rawlings, Nate. "Where Miracles Are Made: An Inside Look at the Center for the
Intrepid." *Time*, April 2, 2012. Accessed June 19, 2014. http://nation.time.com
/2012/04/02/where-miracles-are-made-an-inside-look-at-the-center-for-the
-intrepid/.

Reif, Kingston. "Conflict Fuels Iraqi Health Crisis." *Iraq Health Update*. U.K. Med-
facts, 2006. Accessed March 18, 2014. http://psr-la.org/files/iraqupdate
2006copy.pdf.

Roberts, Les, Diyadh Lafta, Richard Garfield, Jamal Khudhairi, and Gilbert Burn-
ham. "Mortality before and after the 2003 Invasion of Iraq: Cluster Sample
Survey." *Lancet* 364 (2004): 1857–64.

Ronell, Avital. *Crack Wars: Literature-Addiction-Mania*. Lincoln: University of Ne-
braska Press, 1992.

Roos, Robert. "Signs of Tularemia Agent Detected in Houston Air." University of
Minnesota, Center for Infectious Disease Research and Policy, October 10,
2003. Accessed July 10, 2014. http://www.cidrap.umn.edu/news-perspective
/2003/10/signs-tularemia-agent-detected-houston-air.

Rozen, Laura. "The Anthrax Vaccine Scandal." *Salon*, October 14, 2001. Accessed
July 1, 2015. http://www.salon.com/2001/10/15/anthrax_vaccine/.

Rubin, John, director. *The Living Weapon*. 2007.

Schott, Linda. *Reconstructing Women's Thoughts: The Women's International League for
Peace and Freedom before World War II*. Palo Alto: Stanford University Press, 1997.

Schumpeter, Joseph A. *Capitalism, Socialism, and Democracy*. New York: Harper and
Row, 1942.

Schwartz, Jason. "A Brand-New Kick: How an MIT Spinoff Is Revolutionizing Prosthetics." *Boston Magazine*, December 2013. Accessed May 29, 2014. http://www

.bostonmagazine.com/health/article/2013/11/26/prosthetics-research-boston
-biom-ankle-prosthetic/.

Schwartz, Nelson D. "Rumsfeld's Growing Stake in Tamiflu." CNN Money, October 31, 2005. Accessed January 4, 2016. http://money.cnn.com/2005/10/31
/news/newsmakers/fortune_rumsfeld/.

————. "The Tamiflu Tug of War." Fortune, November 14, 2005. Accessed January 4,
2016. http://archive.fortune.com/magazines/fortune/fortune_archive/2005
/11/14/8360685/index.htm.

Schweik, Susan M. The Ugly Laws: Disability in Public. New York: New York University Press, 2009.

Sedgwick, Eve. Touching Feeling: Affect, Pedagogy, Performativity. Durham, N.C.:
Duke University Press, 2002.

Serkin, F., D. Soderdahl, J. Hernandez, M. Patterson, L. Blackbourne, and C. Wade.
"Combat Urologic Trauma in U.S. Military Overseas Contingency Operations."
Journal of Trauma 69 (2010): S175–78.

Serlin, David. "Disability, Masculinity, and the Prosthetics of War, 1945–2005." In
The Prosthetic Impulse: From a Posthuman Present to a Biocultural Future, ed. Marquard Smith and Joanna Morra, 155–86. Cambridge, Mass.: MIT Press, 2006.

————. "Queerness and Disability in U.S. Military Culture." GLQ 9.1–2 (2003):
149–79.

————. Replaceable You: Engineering the Body in Postwar America. Chicago: University of Chicago Press, 2004.

Shakespeare, Tom. Disability Rights and Wrongs Revisited. 2nd ed. London: Routledge, 2014.

Shea, Dana A. "The National Biodefense Analysis and Countermeasures Center: Issues for Congress." Congressional Research Service Report, February 15, 2007.

SIGIR. "January 2006: Quarterly Report to Congress." Accessed March 20, 2014.
http://cybercemetery.unt.edu/archive/sigir/20131001093125/http://www
.sigir.mil/publications/quarterlyreports/January2006.html.

Sisk, Richard. "DoD: 5,000 Military Families Losing Food Stamps." Military.com,
July 13, 2013. Accessed June 9, 2015. http://www.military.com/daily-news
/2013/07/13/dod-5000-military-families-losing-food-stamps.html.

Skocpol, Theda. Protecting Soldiers and Mothers: The Political Origins of Social Policy
in the United States. Cambridge, Mass.: Harvard University Press, 1992.

Smith, Amelia. "Polio-Related Murders Kill More than Disease Itself." Newsweek,
November 28, 2014. Accessed June 15, 2015. http://europe.newsweek.com
/polio-related-murders-kill-more-disease-itself-287880.

Smith, Marquard, and Joanne Morra, eds. The Prosthetic Impulse: From a Posthuman
Present to a Biocultural Future. Cambridge, Mass.: MIT Press, 2006.

Solnit, Rebecca. A Paradise Built in Hell: The Extraordinary Communities That Arise in
Disaster. New York: Penguin Books, 2009.

Spiro, Ellen, and Phil Donahue. Body of War. Documentary film. 2007. http://www
.bodyofwar.com/.

Stewart, Kathleen. *Ordinary Affects*. Durham, N.C.: Duke University Press, 2007.

———. "Worlding: Emergent Forms and the Futures They Project." Presentation at the University of Kentucky, 2015.

Swerdlow, Amy. *Women Strike for Peace*. Chicago: University of Chicago Press, 1993.

Terry, Jennifer. "Significant Injury: War, Medicine, and Empire in Claudia's Case." *Women's Studies Quarterly* 37.1–2 (2009): 220–25.

Ticktin, Miriam. *Casualties of Care: Immigration and the Politics of Humanitarianism in France*. Berkeley: University of California Press, 2011.

Tucker, Jonathan B. "Biological Threat Assessment: Is the Cure Worse than the Disease?" *Arms Control Today*, October 2004.

Underwood, Anne. "Military Medicine: The War on Wounds." *Newsweek*, May 10, 2008. Accessed June 20, 2012. http://www.newsweek.com/military-medicine -war-wounds-90119.

U.S. Army. "Special Compensation for Assistance with Activities of Daily Living (SCAADL)." *My Army Benefits*. Accessed February 20, 2012. http://myarmy benefits.us.army.mil/Home/Benefit_Library/Federal_Benefits_Page/Special _Compensation_for_Assistance_with_Activities_of_Daily_Living_%28SCAADL %29.html?serv=148.

U.S. Army. Center for Army Lessons Learned. "Commander's Guide to Biometrics in Afghanistan: Observations, Insights, and Lessons." Handbook No. 11-25. April 2011. Accessed June 15, 2015. https://info.publicintelligence.net/CALL -AfghanBiometrics.pdf.

U.S. Army. Dismounted Complex Blast Injury Task Force. Report. Fort Sam Houston, Texas, June 18, 2011. Accessed June 10, 2014. http://armymedicine.mil /Documents/DCBI-Task-Force-Report-Redacted-Final.pdf.

U.S. Army. *Field Manual 3-0, Operations*. June 14, 2001. Accessed February 26, 2017. http://www.globalsecurity.org/military/library/policy/army/fm/3-0/index .html.

U.S. Army and Marine Corps. *Counterinsurgency: Field Manual 3-24*. Boulder: Paladin Press, 2007.

U.S. Centers for Disease Control and Prevention. "H5 Viruses in the United States." Accessed January 3, 2016. http://www.cdc.gov/flu/avianflu/h5/.

———. "Progress toward Poliomyelitis Eradication—Pakistan, January 2012–September 2013." *Morbidity and Mortality Weekly Report*, November 22, 2013, 934–38. Accessed June 15, 2015. http://www.cdc.gov/mmwr/preview/mmwrhtml /mm6246a6.htm.

———. "The 2009 H1N1 Pandemic: Summary Highlights, April 2009–April 2010." June 16, 2010. Accessed August 1, 2016. http://www.cdc.gov/h1n1flu/cdc response.htm.

———. "What Are the Signs and Symptoms of Concussion?" Accessed April 10, 2014. http://www.cdc.gov/concussion/signs_symptoms.html.

U.S. Congress. *Final Report of the Select Committee to Study Governmental Operations with Respect to Intelligence Activities, Foreign and Military Intelligence*. Report

No. 94-755. 94th Cong., 2d Sess. Washington, D.C.: U.S. Government Printing Office, 1976.

———. "Is Military Research Hazardous to Veterans' Health? Lessons Spanning Half a Century." Staff Report prepared for the Committee on Veterans' Affairs, December 8, 1994. 103rd Congress, 2d Sess. *Gulf War Vets*. Accessed December 20, 2016. http://www.gulfwarvets.com/senate.htm.

———. Pandemic and All-Hazards Preparedness Act (S.3678). 109th Congress. *Govtrack*, December 14, 2006. Accessed July 23, 2015. https://www.govtrack.us/congress/bills/109/s3678/text.

U.S. Congressional Budget Office. "The Veterans Health Administration's Treatment of PTSD and Traumatic Brain Injury among Recent Combat Veterans." February 2012. Accessed April 10, 2014. http://www.cbo.gov/sites/default/files/cbofiles/attachments/02-09-PTSD.pdf.

U.S. Department of Commerce. Census Bureau. "Age by Veteran Status by Poverty Status in the Past 12 Months by Disability Status for the Civilian Population 18 Years and Over, 2008–2010." Accessed June 9, 2015. http://factfinder.census.gov/faces/tableservices/jsf/pages/productview.xhtml?pid=ACS_10_3YR_C21007&prodType=table.

U.S. Department of Defense. News Briefing, Secretary Rumsfeld and General Richard Myers. February 12, 2002. Accessed February 26, 2017. http://archive.defense.gov/Transcripts/Transcript.aspx?TranscriptID=2636.

———. News Transcript. Secretary Rumsfeld Press Conference at NATO Headquarters, Brussels, Belgium. June 6, 2002. Accessed February 26, 2017. http://www.nato.int/docu/speech/2002/s020606g.htm.

———. *Quadrennial Defense Review Report*. Washington, D.C.: U.S. Government Printing Office, 2010.

U.S. Department of Homeland Security. "If You See Something, Say Something™." Accessed January 8, 2014. https://www.dhs.gov/see-something-say-something.

U.S. Department of Housing and Urban Development. Office of Community Planning and Development. "The 2011 Point-in-Time Estimates of Homelessness: Supplement to the Annual Assessment Report." December 2011. Accessed June 9, 2015. https://www.hudexchange.info/resources/documents/PIT-HIC_SupplementalAHARReport.pdf.

U.S. Department of Veterans Affairs. "Annual Benefits Report Fiscal Year 2012." Accessed June 9, 2015. http://www.va.gov/budget/docs/report/archive/FY-2011_VA-PerformanceAccountabilityHighlights.pdf.

———. "Frequently Asked Questions." Accessed April 4, 2014. http://www.polytrauma.va.gov/faq.asp?FAQ#FAQ2.

———. "Polytrauma/TBI System of Care." Accessed April 25, 2014. http://www.polytrauma.va.gov.

U.S. Department of Veterans Affairs. Office of Public and Intergovernmental Affairs. "VA Conducts Nation's Largest Analysis of Veteran Suicide." July 7, 2016.

Accessed July 17, 2016. http://www.va.gov/opa/pressrel/pressrelease.cfm
?id=2801.

———. "VA-HUD: Homelessness among Veterans Declines 12% in 2011." December 13, 2011. Accessed June 9, 2015. http://www.va.gov/opa/pressrel/press
release.cfm?id=2234.

U.S. House of Representatives. "H. Rept. 109-746: Report on Activities During the
109th Congress." 109th Congress (2005–2006). January 2, 2007. Accessed
July 21, 2015. https://www.congress.gov/congressional-report/109th-congress
/house-report/746/1.

U.S. Senate. "Avian Flu Pandemic." Transcripts of the Senate proceedings on
September 29, 2005 concerning Amendment No. 1886 to the Department of
Defense Appropriations Act, 2006, Volume 151, No. 124, Congressional Record
S10656, pp. S10653–S10692. Accessed February 26, 2017. https://www.congress
.gov/congressional-record/2005/09/29/senate-section/article/S10652-2.

Venkataramanan, Madhumita. "In Pictures: The Biomechatronics of MIT." *Wired
UK*, November 12, 2012. Accessed June 26, 2014. http://www.wired.co.uk
/magazine/archive/2012/11/features/giant-steps.

Virilio, Paul. *The Vision Machine*. Bloomington: Indiana University Press, 1994.

Wald, Priscilla. *Contagious: Cultures, Carriers, and the Outbreak Narrative*. Durham,
N.C.: Duke University Press, 2008.

Warden, Deborah. "Military TBI during the Iraq and Afghanistan Wars." *Journal of
Head Trauma and Rehabilitation* 21.5 (2006): 398–402.

Washington, Harriet A. *Medical Apartheid: The Dark History of Medical Experimentation on Black Americans from Colonial Times to the Present*. New York: Anchor
Books, 2006.

Watson Institute for International and Public Affairs, Brown University. "Afghan
Civilians." *Costs of War*. Accessed February 26, 2017. http://watson.brown.edu
/costsofwar/costs/human/civilians/afghan.gregory.

Waxman, Steve. "War and Male Genital Trauma." *American Fertility Association*,
March 15, 2012. Accessed April 9, 2014. http://www.theafa.org/article/war-and
-male-genital-trauma/.

Waxman, Steve, A. Beekely, A. Morey, and D. Soderdahl. "Penetrating Trauma to
the External Genitalia in Operation Iraqi Freedom." *International Journal of
Impotence Research* 21.2 (2009): 145–48.

Weizman, Eyal. *The Least of All Possible Evils: Humanitarian Violence from Arendt to
Gaza*. London: Verso, 2011.

Wessberg, J., C. R. Stambaugh, J. D. Kralik, P. D. Beck, M. Laubach, J. K. Chapin, J.
Kim, S. J. Biggs, M. A. Srinivasan, and M. A. Nicolelis. "Real-Time Prediction
of Hand Trajectory by Ensembles in Cortical Neurons in Primates." *Nature* 408
(2000): 361–65.

Wheelis, Mark, Lajos Rózsa, and Malcolm Dando, eds. *Deadly Cultures: Biological
Weapons since 1945*. Cambridge, Mass.: Harvard University Press, 2006.

Whitehead, Gregory. "Display Wounds." June 7, 2012. Accessed May 12, 2014. http://gregorywhitehead.net/2012/06/07/display-wounds/.

———. "Display Wounds: Rumination of a Vulnerologist." In *When Pain Strikes Back: Theory Out of Bounds*, ed. Bill Burns, Cathy Busby, and Kim Sawchuck, 133–40. Minneapolis: University of Minnesota Press, 1999.

White House. "Critical Infrastructure Protection." PDD/NSC-63. May 22, 1998. Federation of American Scientists. Accessed July 28, 2015. https://fas.org/irp/offdocs/pdd/pdd-63.htm.

———. "Fact Sheet: The New Way Forward in Iraq." January 2007. Accessed February 26, 2017. https://georgewbush-whitehouse.archives.gov/news/releases/2007/01/20070110-3.html.

———. "Protection against Unconventional Threats to the Homeland and Americans Overseas." PDD/NSC-62. May 22, 1998. Federation of American Scientists. Accessed July 28, 2015. https://fas.org/irp/offdocs/pdd/pdd-62.pdf.

———. "Remarks of President Barack Obama as Prepared for Delivery Signing of Stem Cell Executive Order [EO 13505] and Scientific Integrity Memorandum." March 9, 2009. Accessed May 1, 2014. http://www.whitehouse.gov/the_press_office/Remarks-of-the-President-As-Prepared-for-Delivery-Signing-of-Stem-Cell-Executive-Order-and-Scientific-Integrity-Presidential-Memorandum.

———. "The 2003 State of the Union Address: Complete Transcript of President Bush's Speech to Congress and the Nation." January 28, 2003. Accessed July 21, 2015. http://whitehouse.georgewbush.org/news/2003/012803-SOTU.asp.

———. "U.S. Policy on Counterterrorism." PDD/NSC-39. July 21, 1995. Federation of American Scientists. Accessed July 28, 2015. https://fas.org/irp/offdocs/pdd39.htm.

Wibben, Annick T. R. *Feminist Security Studies: A Narrative Approach*. London: Routledge, 2011.

Williams, Sean. "Five Unlikely Companies Bucking the Biotech Sell-Off." *Motley Fool*, April 15, 2014. Accessed May 12, 2014. http://www.fool.com/investing/general/2014/04/15/5-unlikely-companies-bucking-the-biotech-sell-off.aspx.

Wolbring, Gregor. "Disability Rights Approach toward Bioethics." *Journal of Disability Policy Studies* 14.3 (2003): 174–80.

Wool, Zoë. *After War: The Weight of Life at Walter Reed*. Durham, N.C.: Duke University Press, 2015.

———. "On Movement: The Matter of U.S. Soldiers' Being after Combat." *Ethnos: Journal of Anthropology* 78.3 (2013): 1–31.

World Health Organization. "Republic of Iraq: Iraq Family Health Survey Report." January 9, 2008. Accessed March 18, 2014. http://www.who.int/mediacentre/news/releases/2008/pr02/2008_iraq_family_health_survey_report.pdf.

World Health Organization and UN Children's Fund. Countdown to 2015: Maternal, Newborn, and Child Survival. "Afghanistan." 2012. Accessed March 19, 2014. http://www.countdown2015mnch.org/documents/2012Report/2012/2012_Afghanistan.pdf.

INDEX

Abbottabad, Pakistan, 49
Abrams, Elliott, 160
Addams, Jane, 183
Affordable Care Act of 2010, 16
Afghan civilians: absence from biomedical salvation stories, 24, 63,
88, 178; catastrophic displacement,
24, 46; compensation for losses, 51,
197n61; counterinsurgency operations, 39–42; deaths, 22, 51; health
care system, 42, 45–46; and neoliberalism, 45–46; women, 40–42;
wounded, 22, 24, 46, 88, 139, 178
Afghanistan: catastrophic violence,
48; counterinsurgency operations,
40–42; rebuilding of, 22, 42, 45;
returning veterans, 21, 54, 58, 63,
69, 90, 92, 89, 102, 110, 123–24,
129, 192n25, 193n33, 198n14; Soviet
intervention in, 153; troop surge
of 2009, 38; U.S. occupation of, 17,
28, 34, 46–47, 50; war, 2, 4, 8, 22,
58, 90
AFIRM. *See* Armed Forces Institute of
Regenerative Medicine
Afridi, Shakil, 48–49
Agent Orange, 155
Ahuja, Neel, 143
Alzheimer's disease, 79
American Civil Liberties Union (ACLU),
183, 193n33
American Enterprise Institute, 160

American Medical Association, 178
amputees, 4, 14, 25, 69, 89–90, 93, 99,
101, 108–10, 112, 121, 124, 127, 129,
130, 133–36, 220n31, 207n64
amyotrophic lateral sclerosis, 79
Anderson, Chris, 116
anthrax: attacks of 2001, 68, 141–42,
144–45, 160–61, 167, 170, 173–77,
200n27; deaths from, 174; Department of Defense vaccine program,
154–59; exposure to, 164; mock
attacks, 171; Saudi Arabian vaccine
purchase, 158; types of, 156; vaccination manufacturing, 167–68
Anthrax Vaccine Adsorbed (AVA), 154,
156
Anthrax Vaccine Immunization Program (AVIP), 155
antibiotics, 5, 20, 161, 166, 174, 178
antivirals, 5, 161
Armed Forces Institute of Regenerative
Medicine (AFIRM), 53, 74–77, 80–81,
197n1, 201n38
Army Center for Enhanced Performance, 64
artificial intelligence, 5, 7, 57, 91, 93–94,
101, 106–7
Atala, Anthony, 54, 65–68, 81–82
attachment theory, 11, 188, 191n13
attention-deficit disorder, 118
avian flu, 140–41, 145, 148, 165, 175–76,
208n1

Ba'ath Party, 43
Badylak, Stephen, 68–69
Bagram Airfield, 16
Basic Package of Health Services
(BPHS), 45
Bell, Colleen, 36, 39
Benanav, Aaron, 24
Benard, Cheryl, 42
benevolence, 39, 124, 146, 181, 188
Bennett, Jane, 101
Bennett, William J., 160
Berlant, Lauren, 14, 92, 191n15
Bezos, Jeff, 117
biblical passages, 18, 175, 215n9
Bill and Melinda Gates Foundation,
148
bin Laden, Osama, 48
bio-inequality, 20–21, 50. *See also* unequal economy of life
Biological and Toxin Weapons Convention (BTWC), 152, 160, 162, 163
biological warfare, 5, 26, 146–47, 151–
54, 160–62, 166, 170–71, 173
biological weapons, 34, 122, 142–45,
150–54, 171–72, 174–75, 213–14n63
Biomedical Advanced Research and
Development Authority (BARDA),
145, 164–65, 168–69
biomedical industry, 5, 7, 12, 21, 24,
142, 188. *See also* bionics: industry;
biotechnology: industry
biomedicalization, 25, 95
biomedical logics, 3–4, 7, 27–28, 34, 54–
55, 91–92, 142, 147, 180–81, 188
biomedical salvation, 6, 9, 15–20, 24–25,
52, 54–55, 64–66, 69, 73, 78, 86–87,
90–91, 97, 111, 125, 137–38, 147,
178, 186, 188. *See also* technological
salvation
biomedical war-profiteering, 7, 142, 149,
156, 167
biomedicine, 3, 7, 10, 21; and disposable
life, 24–25, 28, 34, 170; enchantment

with, 4–5, 87; humanitarian, 149,
210n17; militarized, 28, 35; as salve
for violence, 15
biomedicine-war nexus, 4–6, 12, 14,
19–20, 24–25, 27, 51, 56, 73, 180, 187
bionics: defined, 92; design, 4, 90;
devices, 5–6, 19, 25, 89, 91, 93, 95,
99–102, 106, 110, 114–16, 118–20, 124,
126, 129, 137–39; ethical uses of, 132;
industry, 98; neural, 90, 101, 135, 138;
neurons, 112; personal, 108–9, 111;
salvation, 118; science, 113
Bionic Woman, The, 92, 102
biopolitics, 3, 23, 32, 51, 88, 143
BioPort, Inc., 155–59, 167–68
biotechnology, 25, 87, 89, 105, 149, 168;
federal funding for, 145; industry, 4,
7, 19, 55, 65, 76–77, 122, 142, 151, 155,
158, 161, 166, 175–76, 208n9; market
for, 23, 26, 167, 212n52
Blackwell, Joyce, 183
blast injuries, 57–63, 82–83, 89, 118, 120,
128, 133, 198–99n14. *See also* genital
injuries; polytrauma
blood-banking, 14, 99
blood-clotting products, 6, 58, 65
Bolton, John, 160
Boston Marathon bombing, 100, 118,
120, 206–7n53
botulism, 168, 171
Bowlby, John, 11, 191n13
brain-machine interface (BMI), 100,
111, 134, 203n16
Bratton, Benjamin, 117–18
Bremer, J. Paul, 23
Brin, Sergey, 117
Brokaw, Tom, 200n27
Burkle, Frederick, Jr., 44
burn injuries, 57, 61, 65, 69, 79–80, 110,
131
Burr, Richard, 141, 145, 165
Bush, George H. W., 152, 157
Bush, George W., 2, 13, 17–19, 22–23, 32,

35, 42–43, 47–48, 50, 62, 67, 74, 140, 142, 144–45, 152, 160–61, 163, 165, 176

Bush, Vannevar, 30

capitalism: consumer, 94; disaster, 17, 191n21; finance, 19; free-market, 2, 17, 23; industrial, 96, 98; post-Fordist, 98, 138, 203–4n19

care: entangled in war, 4, 7, 19, 24, 39–40, 48, 51, 54, 181, 188; ethic of, 2–3, 27–28, 54, 91, 106, 125, 146–47, 186

Cartwright, Lisa, 100, 111

Carver Village: Florida, 171–73; Georgia, 172–73

Centers for Disease Control and Prevention (CDC), 49, 140–41, 148, 151, 162, 175–77, 200n27, 214n68

Centre for Applied Microbiology and Research, 156, 158

chemical, biological, radioactive, and nuclear weapons (CBRN), 163. *See also* biological weapons; chemical weapons

chemical weapons, 76, 151, 154, 156, 172

Cheney, Richard, 2, 44, 48, 160

Christianity, 18, 69

CIA: operation in Abbottabad, 48–49; secret experiments of, 171–72, 213n63

citizenship: and military service, 21; status, 20, 157, 189n3

class. *See* socioeconomic class

Clegg, John, 24

Cleveland Clinic, 76, 103, 201n41, 204n27

Clinton, Bill, 153–54, 159–60

Clinton Global Initiative, 148–49

cloning, 79

cluster bombs, 63

Coalition Provisional Authority, 23, 42–45

cochlear implants, 92, 119

Cohen, William S., 154–55, 157

COIN. *See* counterinsurgency

Cold War, 10, 13, 16, 30–31, 142, 152–53, 161, 213n63

collateral damage, 35, 50–51

colonial feminism, 40

colonialism, 29, 39; of the mind, 29, 39, 143

condolence payments, 193n33

contamination, 97, 153, 156, 162, 173

counterinsurgency (COIN): doctrine of, 28, 36, 38; gender strategies of, 39–42; as medical interventions, 36–39; operations, 27, 51, 62, 147

countermeasures. *See* medical countermeasures

counterterror state, 141–42, 144, 149–50, 174, 178

Crawford, Cassandra, 101, 130

Crowe, William, 157

cruel optimism, 14, 52, 54, 65, 92, 188

Culp, Connie, 204n27

cultural studies, 8

daisy cutter bombs, 63

Dalai Lama, 105

DARPA. *See* Defense Advanced Research Projects Agency

Daschle, Tom, 200n27

Deaf culture, 119

debt, 5, 13, 18–20, 24, 47, 72–73, 83, 87, 91, 96, 106, 123, 125, 130, 137

Defense Advanced Research Projects Agency (DARPA), 89, 91, 104, 106, 123–25, 127, 130, 134, 161, 201n38, 203n16, 205n33; Biological Technologies Office, 90, 122; Human Assisted Neural Hand Devices program, 123; Revolutionizing Prosthetics program, 90, 121, 122

DEKA Arm, 124, 127–29, 133

DEKA Research and Development Corporation, 126

dengue fever, 172

Department of Defense: anthrax vaccination program, 154–55, 157–59; biosecurity program, 166, 170; controversy over using experimental drugs, 173; funded research, 64–65, 98, 108, 111; and humanitarian aid, 43, 208n1; and nation-building, 44

Department of Health and Human Services (HHS), 164, 168–70

Department of Homeland Security (DHS): biosecurity programs of, 145, 161–64; citizen surveillance programs, 32–33. See also homeland security

Department of Veterans Affairs, 59, 109, 173, 197n1

depression, 11, 114, 118, 175

destroy-and-build logic, 7, 17, 27, 42–43, 48, 187

diabetes, 79, 138, 190n5

Dick, Philip K., 105

disability rights, 113, 119, 206n52

disability studies, 8, 94–95, 119

dismounted complex blast injury (DCBI), 57, 61–62, 198–99n14. See also genital injuries

Disney Corporation, 105

Doctors without Borders, 46, 182

doctrine of counterproliferation, 151, 153–54

domestic terrorism, 68, 153, 173

Donoghue, John, 111, 114

Dorrance, David, 121

Dorrance hook, 122, 133–34

Downs, Fred, 124, 128–29

Dreyfuss, Henry, 100

drones: attacks, 4, 49; and targeted assassinations, 19, 35. See also unmanned aerial vehicles

Duke University, 123, 128, 133, 208–9n9

Ebola virus, 145, 148

economization of life, 23, 48

Einstein, Alfred, 105

Elbe, Stefan, 147

El-Hibri, Fuad, 157–58, 167

El-Hibri, Ibrahim, 157–58

embryogenesis, 86

embryology, 78

Emergent BioSolutions, 167–69, 177

empire, 30; U.S., 4, 18, 86, 143, 186

Enriquez, Juan, 117

environmental damage, 5, 179, 181–82, 185

Environmental Protection Agency (EPA), 154, 162, 185

epidemiology, 143, 150

Essential Package of Hospital Services (EPHS), 45

ethnic studies, 8

evacuation procedures, 6, 58, 65, 86

everyday life, 4, 125; disciplining of citizens in, 10; militarization of, 27–29, 51

extracellular matrix (ECM), 68–70

face transplants, 103, 204–5n27

Fanon, Frantz, 39

FBI: anthrax investigation, 141; biosecurity programs, 162

Female Engagement Teams (FET), 41–42

femininity, 84

feminist organizations, 184–85

feminist science studies, 8–9

fetuses, 68, 73–74, 78–81, 85

financial speculation, 5–6, 22, 26, 32, 87, 146, 154, 212n52

Food and Drug Administration (FDA), 127, 159

food stamps, 192–93n27

Ford, Gerald, 160, 213n63

Fort Detrick, Maryland, 171, 175, 214n63

Foucault, Michel, 7, 32, 51

Garfield, Richard, 44

Garland-Thomson, Rosemary, 96–97

Gates, Bill, 117

gender: and counterinsurgency strategies, 39–41; hierarchies of, 108; ideologies of, 86, 91, 104, 183; and rehabilitation, 84, 85; as a social technology, 6, 8, 20

genital injuries, 62, 81–83, 85, 198n12, 198n14, 202n50

Ghani, Ashraf, 117

Gilead Sciences, Inc., 175–77

Global War on Terror, 7, 10, 18, 22, 31, 40, 42, 57, 68, 120, 142, 146, 188, 192n25, 213n52

Goldfarb, Brian, 100, 111

Google, 117

Gulf War. *See* Persian Gulf War

H1N1 virus, 170. *See also* avian flu

H5N1 virus, 140–41, 143, 175–77. *See also* avian flu

Hall, Stuart, 8

Hanson, David, 89, 91, 102, 104–8, 205n31

Haraway, Donna J., 9, 181, 186

Harkin, Tom, 140–41, 165, 175–77

Harvard University, 113, 117, 120, 201n41

Haslet-Davis, Adrianne, 119–21

health care: Afghan system, 45, 47; as a basic right, 148; and counterinsurgency, 28, 37, 41–42, 47–48; high cost of, 5, 34, 45, 189–90n5; industry, 16, 42; Iraqi national system, 43; lack of access to, 34, 88, 171; privatization of, 42–43, 45–46; for U.S. veterans, 185, 192n25

health maintenance organization (HMO), 45

heirloom seeds, 23

Helms, Richard, 213n63

Hernandez, Isais, 69–71

Herr, Hugh, 89, 91, 102, 109–16, 118–21, 133–34, 205n36, 206n41, 206n45, 206n48, 220

heteronormativity, 63

heterosexuality: compulsory, 12; and conjugal couple, 84; and masculinity, 85, 87; and nationalism, 86–87; valorization of, 98

HHS. *See* Department of Health and Human Services

Hippocratic Oath, 182

HIV/AIDS, 49, 148–49, 190n5, 203–4n19

Hockenberry, John, 113

homeland security, 27, 29, 32, 137, 145. *See also* Department of Homeland Security

homophobia, 185

Hubbard, Ruth, 9

human capital, 20, 23, 47, 193n34

human genome project, 105, 212n52

Hurricane Katrina, 140, 208n1

Hussein, Saddam: fall of regime, 23, 43, 177; invasion of Kuwait, 158; obstruction of UN weapons inspectors, 157; and weapons of mass destruction, 145, 160

hyphema, 60

IED. *See* improvised explosive device

imperialism, 1, 26, 124, 130, 143, 179–80, 186, 188

improvised explosive device (IED), 6, 57, 61–62, 83, 187, 198n12, 202n50

infectious disease, 5, 13; and bioinequality, 20, 172, 178; efforts to contain, 31, 44, 148–49, 164; metaphor for enemy in war, 35; military research on, 13, 76, 150; production of, 161; weaponizing, 172

influenza. *See* avian flu

International Monetary Fund (IMF), 24, 47, 197n61

International Red Cross, 182

International Relations, 8

intimacy, 24, 83–84, 100–101

Iran-Iraq War (1980–1988), 43

Iraq: catastrophic violence, 48; rebuilding of, 22–23, 42–47; returning

Iraq (*continued*)
veterans, 21, 54, 58, 63, 90, 92, 89, 102, 110, 123–24, 129, 186, 192n25, 198n14; troop surge (2007), 38; U.S. occupation of, 17, 28, 34, 46–47, 50; war, 2, 4, 8, 22, 51, 90, 136, 141, 145, 160, 177; weapons development, 153. *See also* Iraqi civilians; Hussein, Saddam; Persian Gulf War

Iraqi civilians: absence from biomedical salvation stories, 24, 63, 139, 178; catastrophic displacement, 24, 44, 185, 215n7; compensation for losses, 23, 51, 193n33, 197n61; deaths, 22, 51; economic sanctions, 43; farmers, 23; health care system, 42, 44–45; and neoliberalism, 23, 42; physicians, 43–44, 194n34, 196n40; wounded, 22, 24, 44, 46, 88, 139, 178

Iraqi Ministry of Health, 45

Iraq Veterans against the War (IVAW), 185–86, 215n7

Islamic Republic of Afghanistan, 37

Itskov, Dmitry, 105

Ivins, Bruce, 175

Johns Hopkins University, 123, 201n41

Journal of the American Medical Association, 178

Jurgenson, Nathan, 118

Kabul University, 117

Kamen, Dean, 126–28

Kamen, Jack, 126

Kennedy, Ted, 140

Kenny, Katherine E., 47

Khalili, Laleh, 40

Khalilizad, Zalmay, 42

Kinsey, Alfred C., 99

known unknowns, 146, 209n10

Korean War, 1, 10, 183

Kristol, William, 160

Kuiken, Todd, 112, 130–32

Ku Klux Klan, 171

Kuniholm, Jonathan, 128–29, 133–37

Kurzweil, Ray, 117

Kuwait, 158

Lakoff, Andrew, 148–49

Lancet, 46, 51

Leahy, Patrick, 200n27

Li, Tania, 51

Ling, Geoff, 90, 102, 124–26, 129

Linker, Beth, 84

Litynski, Mark, 83

Lockheed Martin, 60–61, 198n11

Lukes, H. M., 95

MAD Magazine, 126

Maeda, John, 117

malaria, 13, 149, 172

Mallon, Mary, 150

Maloney, Joshua, 70–72

Martin, Emily, 203–4n19

Martin, Trayvon, 33

Masco, Joseph, 10, 32, 144

masculinity, 12, 40, 83–85, 87, 96, 98–99

Massachusetts Institute of Technology (MIT), 113, 117, 137, 181, 201n41; Media Lab, 89, 109, 115; H2.0 Symposium, 113–14

McCain, John, 136

McCarthy, Paul, 104–5

McChrystal, Stanley, 41

McGowan Institute (University of Pittsburgh), 68, 201n41

Médecins sans Frontières (MSF). *See* Doctors without Borders

media: industries, 4, 30, 105, 141; narratives, 5, 17–18, 24, 55, 64–65, 73, 83, 135; representations, 7, 19, 31, 48, 54, 63, 85, 90–92, 106, 113, 123, 138, 184; social, 117, 136, 186

Medicaid, 16

medical countermeasures, 7, 34, 141–42, 145–46, 149, 151, 154, 161–67, 169–70, 177

Medicare, 16, 192n25

Smith, Marquard, 94
socioeconomic class, 20, 40, 99, 108; as social technology, 6, 8
South Korea, 78, 155
Spivak, Gayatri, 9
Stanford University, 79–80, 117, 157, 175, 201n41
state-sponsored violence, 4. *See also* policing; war
stem cells, 5, 99; adult, 78; banking of, 79; embryonic, 18, 66–67, 74–75, 78–80
Stewart, Katie, 181, 214n1, 235
Strategic National Stockpile, 141, 146, 168
suicide: among veterans, 15, 65, 87, 124; attacks of 9/11, 10, 31, 144; bombings, 40; of Bruce Ivins, 175; of Isabelle Dinoire, 205n27
surgical: as metaphor for counter-insurgency operations, 35; strikes, 2, 35, 50; techniques, 14, 70, 82, 104, 112, 131
surveillance, 4, 12, 23, 27, 29, 31–32, 40, 44, 86, 143, 145–46, 148, 159, 161, 201n39, 207n53, 210n13
Syria, 49

Tamiflu, 175–76
targeted assassinations, 19, 50–51
TB. *See* tuberculosis
technological salvation, 115, 117, 119, 130, 133, 146, 186–87, 206n52. *See also* biomedical salvation
TED Talks, 6, 91, 93, 106, 108, 114–16, 118, 120, 127, 130, 132, 138; critique of, 116–18
Terasem movement, 105
testosterone, 82
Thatcher, Margaret, 158
therapists, 85; psychological, 6; rehabilitation, 57, 125
Threat Characterization Center, 162–63

Thyphoid Mary. *See* Mallon, Mary
tissue cultivation, 5, 53–54, 57, 65–66, 68–69, 70–73, 77–82, 87, 89, 99, 104. *See also* regenerative medicine; stem cells
Tissue Engineering Regenerative Medicine International Society, 68
torture, 5, 23, 34, 182
Total War Society, 8, 29–31, 51
Transformational Medical Technologies initiative, 166
transnational circuits, 5
traumatic brain injury (TBI), 57–59, 118, 124, 178, 186, 199n16
troop surges: of 2007 in Iraq, 38, 62; of 2009 in Afghanistan, 38, 62
Tsarnaev, Dzhokhar, 207n53
Tsarnaev, Tamerlan, 207n53
tuberculosis, 44, 148–49, 178

"ugly laws," 97
unequal economy of life, 6, 74, 117, 178. *See also* bio-inequality
unknown unknowns, 209n10. *See also* known unknowns
UNICEF, 43
Union of Concerned Scientists, 181
United Therapeutics, 105
University of Pittsburgh, 68, 70, 123, 201n41
University of Texas at Dallas, 105
unmanned aerial vehicles, 50. *See also* drones
U.S. Agency for International Development (USAID), 43–45, 47
USAID. *See* U.S. Agency for International Development
U.S. Army Medical Research and Materiel Command (USAMRMC), 76, 127, 162, 201n39
U.S. Army Telemedicine and Advanced Technology Research Center, 76
U.S. Revolutionary War, 57

VA. *See* Veterans Administration
vaccination programs, 34, 44, 48–49, 148, 157, 174
veterans: of Afghanistan war, 185; bureaucratic inefficiencies suffered by, 21–22, 124, 170; casualty rates, 58; compensation for disabilities, 192n25, 199n17; exposure to toxins, 171, 173; fatality rates, 57; of Iraq War, 185; of Persian Gulf War, 142, 155, 173; and poverty, 21, 192n27; rehabilitation of, 90–93, 101, 125; sacrifices made as attachment to war, 109, 111, 123; suicides of, 15, 65; of Vietnam War, 155, 207n64; of World War I, 102; of World War II, 1, 57, 99; wounded, 12, 17, 25, 53, 56, 62, 64, 72, 78, 82, 86, 96–99, 104, 202n50
Veterans Administration (VA), 22, 58, 64, 75, 98, 100, 111, 124, 170; hospitals, 63, 97, 180. *See also* Department of Veterans Affairs
Veterans for Peace, 185
Victorian culture, 98
video games, 20
Vietnam War, 1, 10, 57, 113, 124, 128, 155, 181, 183–84, 207n64, 215n9
vulnerologist, 55
vulnerology, 60–62

Wake Forest Institute for Regenerative Medicine, 53, 201n41
Wald, Priscilla, 150
Walter Reed Army Institute of Research, 201n39
Walter Reed Army Medical Center, 59, 83, 85, 124–25, 128, 133, 170, 200n31
Walter Reed National Military Medical Center, 53
war: fought in the name of humanity, 3, 6, 14, 22, 50, 180; opposition to, 4,

181, 185; preemptive, 50, 145, 150–51, 160–61, 177; rationalizations for, 2–4, 28, 34–35, 39, 50, 54, 97, 146, 152, 181, 188. *See also* Global War on Terror
war-generated polytrauma, 4
war profiteering, 12, 137, 145
Washington, Harriet, 171–72
weapons of mass destruction (WMD), 31, 34, 142–45, 150, 154, 160, 174
Weird Science, 126
Weizman, Eyal, 50
Whitehead, Gregory, 55
WHO. *See* World Health Organization
whooping cough, 172–73
Wilson, Woodrow, 183
WIRED Magazine, 114
WMD. *See* weapons of mass destruction
Wolfowitz, Paul, 160
Women's International League for Peace and Freedom (WILPF), 182–84
Women Strike for Peace, 183–84
Wood, David, 83
Wool, Zoë, 83–85
World Bank, 23–24, 45, 47, 148
World Health Organization (WHO), 46, 148
World War II, 1, 11, 13, 16, 30, 57, 99, 136, 148, 152, 171, 183, 190n6, 191n13
wound ballistics, 191n6
woundscape, 25, 55, 58–59, 62–63, 86
Wurman, Richard Saul, 116

xenophobia, 10, 27, 143
xenotransplantation, 105

yellow fever, 171–72
Young, Tomas, 186

Zapatistas, 117
Zika virus, 148
Zimmerman, George, 33